BEING POSITIVE

Being Positive

THE LIVES OF
MEN AND WOMEN
WITH HIV

Robert Klitzman, M.D.

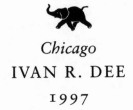

Chicago
IVAN R. DEE
1997

Library of Congress Cataloging-in-Publication Data:
Klitzman, Robert.
Being positive : the lives of men and women with HIV /
Robert Klitzman
p.   cm.
Includes index.
ISBN 1-56663-164-5 (alk. paper)
1. HIV infections—Psychological aspects.   2. HIV-positive persons.
I. Title.
RC607.A26K5755   1997
362.1'969792—dc21   97-16116

To Philip Koether

As if hands were enough
To hold an avalanche off.
—Thom Gunn,
"The Man with Night Sweats"

. . . To state quite simply what we learn in
times of pestilence: that there are more
things to admire in men than to despise.
—Albert Camus, *The Plague*

Contents

Acknowledgments

MANY PEOPLE have helped me with this book. Most important, I am deeply indebted to the men and women I interviewed who shared their experiences with me and let me into their lives. I could not have written this book without their trust and help.

I am also deeply indebted to Renée Fox, who read through all the interviews I conducted and helped me to analyze them. She has been an unfailing mentor and friend, and this book owes much to her generosity and support. At the HIV Center for Clinical and Behavioral Studies at the New York State Psychiatric Institute and the Columbia University Department of Psychiatry I want to thank Robert Kertzner, Mervyn Susser, Anke Ehrhardt, Zena Stein, Ronald Bayer, George Todak, Lucille Newman, and Janet Williams. Funding for this project was provided in part by the National Institutes of Mental Health through the Center (grant P50 MH43520), the postdoctoral behavioral science research training program (grant T32 MH19139), and a career development award (K08 MH01420-01). For assistance with transcribing and typing I am grateful to Roberta Leftenant, Dorothy Lewis, Stacey Spence, and Mitchell Sally.

For institutional support while conducting this research I also wish to thank the Robert Wood Johnson Foundation Clinical Scholars Program at the University of Pennsylvania, and in particular Sankey Williams and the late Samuel Martin.

I am grateful to the Aaron Diamond Foundation Post-Doctoral Research Fellows Program, the Merck Company Foundation, the Corporation of Yaddo where I wrote part of this text, and the Picker-Commonwealth Scholars Program.

For their insights and help I wish to express my appreciation to Robert Jay Lifton, Robert Coles, Susan Jonas, Richard A. Friedman, and Kristine Dahl.

Finally, I am grateful to Ivan R. Dee for his understanding of and faith in this book.

The names and identifying details of the people interviewed in this book have been changed to protect confidentiality.

R. K.

New York City
April 1997

BEING POSITIVE

Preface: *The Last Disco*

THE BUILDING STOOD at the end of the street—the city's edge. Alongside ran a highway hugging the now-abandoned waterfront. Here the city stopped before a wide expanse of river. Waves lapped in the cold wind. I approached the squat building, its old coat of white paint flaking and chipping away to expose worn bricks underneath. I paused, took a deep breath, and entered the building, a New York City residence for people with AIDS.

Suddenly I remembered having been there once before. In the mid-1980s a friend and I had been looking for a place to go dancing and had been directed here. Just inside the entrance, mirrored balls had spun on the ceiling, sweeping glints of red and yellow light across a vast smoky room throbbing with disco music.

Now office partitions subdivided the space, fluorescent lit. Walls of washable semigloss dull yellow paint dripped with memos, announcements, and calendars thumbtacked over one another. A beige metal watercooler stood between secondhand grey filing cabinets and brown metal bookshelves. In the distance a phone rang. Otherwise a hush hung over everything.

As I waited in the small lobby for a patient I had arranged to meet, the elevator doors opened and a thin black man shuffled out

3

in a plaid flannel shirt, loose jeans, and slippers. His hair was jet black, but he had the slow, precarious walk of the very aged. He moved past me to the closed double glass doors at the entrance, rested his arm on the door's horizontal stainless steel handlebar, and stared out. The street was empty. A slender leafless tree on the opposite sidewalk shook in the wind. A plastic bag flew by. The sky was overcast, grey. He stood for several minutes, then turned around and shuffled back to the elevator. The doors opened to admit him and quickly closed again.

I had first witnessed an epidemic several years earlier. In the Eastern Highlands of Papua New Guinea I had conducted research on the medical epidemiology and medical anthropology of kuru, a viral disease that had killed 90 percent of the women and two-thirds of the entire population of the Stone Age Fore group and its neighbors. The virus—an infectious protein virtually identical to that responsible for Creutzfeldt-Jakob disease in man, scrapie in sheep, and most recently Mad Cow disease—had been transmitted there through cannibalistic feasts. When someone died, his or her loved ones consumed the body, exposing themselves to the virus. When these mourners died, they too were eaten, spreading the disease further.

The Fore, I soon saw, desperately sought to make sense of this devastation in their midst, scouring for causes and cures. They blamed sorcerers—at first from nearby hamlets, later from enemy villages farther afield—rather than viruses they had never heard of and that not even Westerners had yet seen. For protection the natives moved their hamlets and erected tall bamboo walls around groups of huts to keep sorcerers out. Yet the epidemic intensified. Still the Fore continued cannibalism, transmitting the virus further, though Westerners, exploring the region for the first time, urged the natives to stop the practice. The disease's incubation periods lasted, I found, up to thirty years or longer. As a result, the tribesmen failed to associate the illness with the behaviors that had spread the virus decades before.

The Fore instead pursued ever newer treatments, flocking to countersorcerers who professed to have cures and reverse countless cases that I as an outsider considered hypochondriacal. Uninfected surrounding groups feared and shunned the Fore because of this presumed evil power. Historically the Fore had traded and intermarried with outsiders. But no longer. Other villages now stayed away.

At the time these responses all seemed curious to me—the irrational products and prejudices of Stone Age minds. Yet the following year, 1981, when I returned to the United States to begin medical school, the first handful of AIDS cases appeared. I had remained interested in how societies dealt with widespread death and had chosen as my mentor, under whom I would conduct research, Dr. Robert Jay Lifton, who had studied Vietnam veterans and survivors of Hiroshima and Nagasaki. He had written about how individuals struggled to incorporate "death in life," and had argued that issues surrounding death have been ignored by depth psychology and social science. These issues desperately needed to be addressed now, in the late twentieth century, given decades of wars, holocausts, and threats of nuclear disaster.

During my medical training, AIDS spread. For the first time in decades a major epidemic swept through the West, and I observed how this "plague" evoked cultural and psychological responses seemingly analogous to those in Papua New Guinea and in situations of massive death I had been studying. Little had I expected these issues suddenly to be played out and writ as large in my own time and place.

The similarities increasingly struck me. On completing my training as a psychiatrist in 1989 I arranged to work in an HIV mental health clinic at a large hospital. There the experiences of HIV-infected men and women impressed me again and again as different from those of other medical and psychiatric patients. They resembled more those I had encountered in New Guinea and had studied with Lifton. Men and women with HIV (Human Immunodeficiency Virus) confronted not only their own illness but the illnesses of countless others—friends, lovers, spouses, siblings, sometimes even parents. HIV was wiping out entire subcultures, not only gay but drug-using. These patients were survivors, too, and participants in larger political, social, cultural, and economic events. They faced not just the resolution of an episode of depression, say, in order to return to a previous life, but far more existential issues: how to make sense of death and dying in themselves and others, and how to incorporate this widespread devastation into the fabric of their ongoing existence.

In the clinic I addressed psychiatric symptoms and prescribed medications. But I began to wonder how exactly HIV-infected men and women confronted death and such new stresses and still managed to find hope. How did individuals—not just those who ventured to a mental health clinic each week—alter and structure their lives and the world around them in order to find strength?

Lifton in his studies had found that human beings, to confront and accept the end of life, universally sought to establish sources of "symbolic immortality"—ways of connecting to something larger than themselves that would continue on after their own deaths. In the face of massive death, he found, people strove to see themselves as alive—and to create form against the chaos and decay around them. In diverse cultures and historical periods, this goal has been achieved through five basic modes—theologically, biologically (through one's offspring), creatively (through one's work or works), through works of nature, and through "experiential transcendence." The cultural anthropologist Ernest Becker had argued that individuals engage in "Denial of Death," but Lifton insisted that people in fact sought ways to come to terms with mortality by transcending it symbolically. In world literature, for example, the hero's quest—for Odysseus, Dante, Hamlet, and King Lear—consists in effect of wandering through realms of the dead in order to confront and make sense of mortality, enabling the hero to direct and define the remainder of his life. The founders of the world's major religions—Buddha, Moses, Jesus, Muhammad—also embarked on journeys to understand human frailty and finitude, and concluded that the human soul does not perish but continues on. Lifton also found that massive death produced feelings of numbness and stasis, relieved by searches for movement and change.

Yet these universal patterns, Lifton argued, blended with cultural and historical forms and individual psychology. How, then, did these patterns differ from or resemble those triggered by HIV, given the new epidemic's specific features and stresses?

Throughout time, few events have shaped individuals and cultures as radically as epidemics. From the plague in Athens to the Black Death, writers as diverse as Thucydides, Pepys, Defoe, and Camus have observed how such widespread disease radically transforms lives and cultures, tearing apart bonds that hold societies together.

The HIV epidemic, I thought, might reveal and reflect much about responses to death and dying in our own time. The numbers alone suggest AIDS' impact. HIV may already infect one to two million Americans and spreads to forty thousand more people each year. AIDS, the disease of our century, has already killed more Americans than the entire Vietnam War, in some geographic areas more than all this century's wars combined. The epidemic—occurring in the 1980s and 1990s as the millennium draws to a close, as baby boomers and their parents age and seek ways of grappling with mortality, and as modern science shatters older frameworks for understanding life and death—has become both a *cause célèbre* and a catalyst for meditations on mortality. Throughout contemporary culture, in films, literature, and art, the epidemic has prompted an outpouring of death imagery, exposing underlying anxieties. Several films and books about vampires and the bubonic plague, for example, may be seen as referring obliquely to AIDS. The epidemic has become as defining and important to current popular culture as the Vietnam War was in the late 1960s, shaped by as well as shaping the culture at large.

Yet HIV clearly differs in several ways from cases of massive death and disaster studied by Lifton and others. HIV is after all a disease, not a war or a bomb—contagious, stigmatized, and commonest among groups marginalized to begin with. Those most affected by HIV, such as gay men, also differ from other groups. For example, they usually have no children to provide biological links to the future. And in many families, children have become infected with HIV from their parents, thus severing such links.

HIV is also heavily stigmatized and raises a series of moral issues in patients' and others' eyes. The Catholic church, political conservatives, and others have long censured homosexuality and sexual freedom, and drug abuse is considered a scourge by almost all of American society. As a result, many HIV-infected individuals feel they have done something "wrong" by being gay, or "too promiscuous," or using drugs in the first place.

Many patients in the HIV mental health clinic felt HIV constituted "punishment" for their "sins." "I know I shouldn't feel this way," one gay man told me. "But I do." Some issues festered, unresolved—low self-esteem following decades of homophobia, and guilt and anger about having contracted the disease. The specific risks patients took made them feel potentially culpable. Patients consequently struggled to make sense of the devastation around them in moral terms, frequently seeking to assign blame. I treated such individuals with psychotherapy. Yet their feelings often remained strong, tied to moral and spiritual beliefs they had been raised with. Susan Sontag had written in the first decade of the epidemic that the prevalent metaphor of AIDS among the public at large involved stigma. Yet it remained unclear how infected individuals themselves viewed and dealt with these problems of marginalization and rejection, and whether other metaphors had arisen now, given changes in the epidemic.

Responses to other stigmatized conditions have been described classically by the sociologist Erving Goffman. Individuals, he wrote, must learn to manage a "spoiled" social or personal identity by conceptualizing it and controlling who knows of it. Some try to conceal symbols of the condition and "pass"; others "go public." A process of experiences and of changes in the conception of the self results in a "moral career."

Those with HIV must also manage prejudice and their own fear that discovery of their positive HIV status could jeopardize their jobs, homes, and relationships. Yet HIV differs from other sources of stigma examined by Goffman: it is fatal, transmitted through behaviors that are themselves taboo, and occurs after individuals have already struggled for years with stigma and stress from homosexuality, drug abuse, or poverty.

AIDS is also a new disease, without a cure. As with kuru in New Guinea, it has been met with uncertainty, helplessness, and over time a desperate search for solutions and effective remedies. Many with HIV have spent large sums on herbs and alternative non-Western treatments and are skeptical of the health care system.

In short, HIV raises new and challenging issues not simply psychological but social, theological, political, medical, and epistemological.

New issues and debates about the virus are continually emerging. The sociodemographic profile of the epidemic has shifted, with the sharpest rise in new cases now occurring not among gay men but women. The largest overall number of current patients is now found among injecting drug users (or IDU's) and their sexual partners. New government recommendations that all pregnant women be tested for HIV at delivery will identify even higher numbers of female cases. Increasingly, those infected with HIV also contend with poverty. Yet the epidemic marches on in the gay community as well, with younger gay men in particular becoming infected at rising and alarming rates.

Recently the overall number of deaths from AIDS has declined nationally (though it is rising among women). Yet the number of new cases of infection continues to rise by thousands each year. People are still becoming infected but are living longer. Life expectancy has risen largely as a result of improved treatment. Advances have come first with AZT (azidothymidine) and increased clinical experience in the use of prophylactic medications such as Bactrim, then with combinations of antiviral treatments such as ddI (dideoxyinosine) and ddC (dideoxycytidine), and most recently with a new class of drugs called protease inhibitors. The disease has thus progressively become more chroniclike. As a result, it has become more important to understand how individuals can "live with" the illness for many years.

At present, despite press reports heralding advances in combating the disease, many patients remain cautious. Protease inhibitors, for example, appear to offer great hope, but they have unknown side effects and their long-term benefits and ideal use are unclear. Will individuals need to take these drugs for the rest of their lives? What will happen if patients decide to stop? Will relapses occur? These medications must be taken on complicated regimens several times a day. Failure to adhere rigidly to these schedules will lead to the development of resistant strains of virus that could in turn be spread to others, endangering public health. Past claims of HIV treatment breakthroughs that later proved disappointing are a reason for care. Protease inhibitors have already proven ineffective for ten thousand to twenty thousand HIV-infected Americans. Many physicians also misprescribe and fail to monitor properly the new drugs that are rapidly being released on the market. Moreover, these medications remain extremely expensive—approximately $15,000 to $20,000 per person each year. Although some patients have insurance to cover this cost, others have coverage for only a portion of the expense, or lack insurance altogether. Many middle-class patients are particularly stuck—they earn too much to be eligible for Medicaid but have insurance that reimburses only a fraction of the cost and requires the rest to be paid out-of-pocket.

Although the media have presented selected upbeat patients over the course of the epidemic, many of those I saw (both before and since the advent of protease inhibitors) displayed far more distress and uncertainty. To achieve resilience, dignity, and grace, and overcome rage, given the multiple losses resulting from HIV, remains extremely difficult, for some almost impossible. The HIV community, attempting to alter perceptions of the disease as "instant death," has through the years mounted extensive public relations campaigns, with advertisements showing famous people and attractive models "living with the virus." The public too has been pleased to hear that individuals can adapt to the illness.

Yet if everyone were dealing well with HIV, the virus would not continue to spread as rapidly as it is. Each year thousands of people become newly infected by HIV, each exposed by another infected person. Many of those already infected presumably have had difficulty altering their behavior in response to the virus. If they better accepted the illness and integrated it more fully into their lives, they might be more careful in practicing safer sex and in not sharing needles, and thus would not spread the virus to others as frequently (though the uninfected need to protect themselves too). Some patients, caving into despair and angst, resent glossy ads and articles implying that they can or should be upbeat. "How can I 'live with AIDS'?" one man asked me. "It's still killing me. People who tell me, 'Live with it' are really saying, 'Don't bother me about it.' They just don't want to hear about it."

In short, despite reports in the media and in medical journals, much about the disease has been ignored or only superficially discussed. Critical questions remain: not whether people can adapt, given these problems with the disease, but who does, and how exactly? What specific problems do individuals face in their lives, and what patterns of response result? How, specifically, does the virus change inner and outer lives and self-perceptions? How do individuals from different backgrounds confront death, stigma, massive traumas, and uncertainties, yet find meaning and wholeness? How does HIV affect other personal problems? How do people cut through day-to-day and medical concerns to appreciate life more fully and to find strength? What does AIDS reveal about how we can best confront trauma and mortality today?

In the clinic I began to get a sense of these issues, but I saw only how patients presented themselves in my office. I had limited time with them and was pressured to see them in certain ways—in terms of symptoms. How individuals put together their lives, struggled and survived outside the hospital, and found meaning in their lives were essentially ignored by medicine and psychiatry.

Nor has psychosocial research on AIDS adequately addressed these issues. Psychological research, because it has tended to be too quantitative and narrow, has missed much about the epidemic. Investigators have, for example, been surprised and puzzled that individuals with HIV have not been persistently anxious or depressed. Research, using standardized multiple-choice questionnaires that are applied to other psychiatric disorders, has failed to show specifically how patients find solutions to the problems they face. Statistical models attempting to predict, for instance, episodes of unsafe sex, have been far too reductionistic. Issues as complex and nuanced as sexuality, identity, and self-perception call for fuller and richer understandings of people's lives.

These issues have important personal and public health implications. As access to protease inhibitors, proper prescription, and adherence to treatment regimens remain problematic, preventing the further spread of the disease will continue to be crucial. Yet such prevention efforts have not been very effective to date, in large part because we have failed to understand why individuals continue to engage in behaviors that transmit the virus despite their knowledge of the risks. This limitation too stems in turn from a failure to gain a full grasp of individuals' lives—of who they are as people, and how they perceive the issues they confront.

The gap between academic research and the complexity of patients' lives became increasingly and painfully clear to me at professional conferences. Near the close of the Sixth International AIDS Conference in Florence, for example, I found myself in a building located in the distant rear of the conference compound. There hung handmade AIDS quilts—final memorials to individual lives. As I wandered through the huge but deserted hall, ordinarily used as a storage facility, loudspeakers piped in dry academic discussions, droning on about bureaucratic policies concerning the epidemic and the statistical likelihoods of various sexual acts. Amidst the quilts, unmoved and ignored, these remote, disembodied voices fell empty.

It became evermore apparent to me that these critical questions about HIV needed to be addressed and would require interviewing patients of varied backgrounds in-depth, listening closely to language and points of view. In part I was influenced by one of my teachers, the anthropologist Clifford Geertz, who had argued that to understand people in a culture it was vital to study their own perspectives and narratives in order to obtain a "thick description." The psychiatrist Robert Coles has shown as well the importance of listening to individuals in their own words in order to comprehend the complexities of people's moral, political, and religious worlds.

The voices of these patients seem especially important now as the high cost of new medications increasingly widens the gap among the infected, between the rich and poor, the haves and have-nots. Many patients in the HIV mental health clinic, for example, faced HIV as only one of several crises, along with poverty, homelessness, violence, drug abuse, racism, and homophobia. I was constantly amazed by the degree to which physicians in medicine and psychiatry viewed patients in narrow diagnostic categories, ignoring these larger social issues. This problem now grows as a result of managed care, which allows clinicians even less time to spend with patients, and provides patients with even fewer medical and related support services. It is essential to understand the rest of these patients' lives too. The need for this approach with HIV may seem obvious, but, much to my surprise, it had not been systematically undertaken.

The public still commonly perceives those with HIV as "bad" or as deviants—drug users, criminals, and homosexuals. Yet the men and women I met in the clinic struggled to do good. Heightened empathy and understanding could reduce the prejudice and discrimination they face. In addition, films, plays, novels, and other books and essays about HIV have each generally explored only a single individual's story. Larger patterns can only be identified by examining the tales of several people together. These other works have also focused on white middle-class gay men rather than women, African-Americans, Latinos, and injecting drug users, whose experiences must also be heard.

I thus decided to embark on this research and started out one winter afternoon to interview people in the New York City AIDS residence. Until then I had seen patients only in hospital wards and clinics. I left the uptown hospital where I was working and traveled downtown, unsure of what I would find.

I ended up speaking to many residents there, which taught me a great deal. But I began to see how much living in the residence itself shaped their responses. In order to include other individuals, I decided to recruit participants for this study through other means as well. I mailed an advertisement to members of a study of HIV-positive gay men at Columbia University, and placed an ad in a New York City AIDS organization's newsletter. That announcement, I later learned, was cut out and posted on the bulletin boards of other HIV service organizations, as a result of which additional people then contacted me.

Finally, men and women came through word of mouth. Many, hearing about the study from friends who had participated, came, trusting me, having had a friend vouchsafe the experience. I conducted the interviews either in participants' homes and offices or in my office at the hospital, whichever they preferred. I interviewed gay men, and heterosexual men and women. I did not include hemophiliacs, given limited resources. Their situation differs in several regards. None responded to announcements of the study, and HIV no longer spreads among them.

The diversity of those I interviewed turned out to be a marked advantage, enabling me to speak with a broad cross section of people. Any one of these "sites" would have provided a far narrower group. The extraordinary range of these individuals' backgrounds reflects the groups among whom the epidemic continues to increase.

I began the initial session with each participant by posing the same question: When did you first find out your HIV status, and what was your reaction to it at that time? From that, individuals went on, some without a break for over an hour, narrating their experiences. I had developed a list of questions investigating broad areas such as relationships with family members and sexual partners. But surprisingly, most individuals raised these topics on their own in the course of our conversation. In the end I spoke with fifty-four individuals—each twice, one to two weeks apart, for two hours each time. In all, the interviews totaled more than two hundred hours. I have also spent months talking with other patients on these and related issues clinically, and as part of other studies.

The men and women I interviewed expressed their thoughts openly, in part I think because they sensed that I valued what they had to say. When they spoke of spirituality and mortality, I was interested, and they felt I might understand. My training as a psychiatrist helped; I listened, at times encouraging through gesture or word, probing when statements were unclear or when deeper nuances or meanings seemed to lurk. I also drew on my experiences conducting ethnographic research in Papua New Guinea, trying to understand beliefs from individuals' own perspectives rather than my own. In the process these men and women extended me an enormous privilege, permitting me to enter their lives. I tape-recorded the interviews, had the tapes transcribed, and then read and studied the printed texts. Between the two interviews with each participant, I discussed each case with a psychiatric colleague who had extensive clinical expertise on HIV-related issues. I was also extremely fortunate in that Renée Fox, professor of sociology at the University of Pennsylvania and a renowned medical sociologist, agreed to read and analyze the interviews as well. Her input was invaluable. Generally we agreed on the major themes that emerged in each interview. At times she emphasized certain motifs more than I had, and our subsequent discussions clarified the import of certain passages as we came to a consensus. In the end her insights deeply enriched my understanding of the issues that emerged.

Although the details of these individuals' experiences differed, common patterns emerged. The shared issues, crises, meanings (both clinical and cultural), and solutions stood out again and again through the interviews, cutting across lines of class, race, and sexual orientation. Differences emerged too, to be sure. But commonalities remained prominent.

Through these pages I have tried to present a picture—a group portrait—and a sense of the fabric and texture of these individuals' lives. Their stories taught me much about how people find meaning and cope with apparently overwhelming difficulties. From the moment I entered the city AIDS residence and saw the man in the lobby, I sensed I was in a different world. I have tried to convey that world, its landscape and its people, the journey I underwent and what I found there.

The first part of this book presents the problems individuals with HIV face. In essence, these men and women have struggled through several stages not only medically but psychologically and socially, confronting a series of losses—of physical and mental functioning, and of loved ones—that intimate the potential final loss of their own life. Patients (a term I will use loosely, as many don't consider themselves such) also experienced several kinds of rejection—from friends, family, health care workers, and coworkers.

Several patterns of response emerged. First, an alternative culture had arisen—the HIV community or, as some called it, HIV-land—consisting of social organizations and a language of its own. Second, various forms of spirituality provided strength. Third, new forms of work and volunteerism offered meaning and a sense of purpose. Fourth, individuals attempted to reconnect with their families. Fifth, many minimized or reframed their illness in order to deal with it. Sixth, individuals responded to the stresses of HIV by resorting to the use of drugs and alcohol.

These patterns all had implications for mental health and for health behaviors that could potentially transmit the virus to others and impair immune functioning. Beyond the epidemic itself, these responses help us understand how individuals today view and talk about life and death.

To illuminate these themes I decided, following the work of Geertz and others, to draw as directly as possible on the narratives

I heard. Thus I introduce several people briefly and then return to them in greater depth to explore their experiences with regard to particular issues. I believe this approach, in the end, best provides the reader with a sense of each person and of the full range and context of the issues.

Some may feel this book belabors death. AIDS as an embodiment of mortality breeds numbness, analogous to that Lifton found in response to other causes of widespread destruction. But it is important to recognize and confront this psychological defense in ourselves, and not to succumb. One day we will all face our own deaths. The narratives here, illuminating how individuals find insight, strength, and hope, can inspire us all.

I conducted these interviews before the July 1996 International AIDS Conference in Vancouver, when protease inhibitors first began to gain widespread attention and use. Yet my work with HIV-infected patients since then has confirmed that these patterns and underlying themes remain central and are in fact of growing importance as more people are infected with the virus and are living longer.

To orient the reader, the participants' names (all pseudonyms) are listed below, in order of their appearance in the text.

Gay men:

Todd Crenshaw
Roy Gifford
Kerry Musgrove
Maurice Bradford
Aaron Eliot
Ken Landers
Raoul Rodriquez
George Sullivan

Matt Winchell
Roger Babson
Leonard Barber
Jason Gillian
Robert Banoff
Arthur Williams
Tony Wilmot

Heterosexual men:

Reynaldo Fernandez	Rodney Jones
Alfie Montoya	Gary Stevens
Eddie Lourdes	Calvin Taylor
Gregory Colson	Donny Sotelo
Mitchell Walters	

Heterosexual women:

Wilma Smith	Jill Montgomery
Jenny Singer	Dede Alwin
Yvette Bing	Gloria Higgens
Olana Ramirez	Carrie Serano
Lorraina Ortiz	Audrey Baker
Gerry Galvez	Elsa Diaz
Arlene Chambers	Beatrice Rosaro

Part I: PROBLEMS

ONE

Roller Coasters:
Stages and Losses of HIV

A SERIES OF LOSSES marks the course of HIV infection. Patients struggle to cope not only with the virus but with its consequences, each of which hints of further change. As a result, adaptation to HIV occurs not all at once but over time, as a process consisting of stages. Individuals vary as to when they first begin to deal with the virus and in their responses to each of these later junctures.

So My Ears Can Hear What My Mouth Has to Say

Wilma Smith illustrates several of the stages of this journey.

"I still can't believe it," she told me, sitting in my office, shaking her head. A tall, svelte, forty-one-year-old African-American woman, she was wearing an elegant black-and-white checked dress with shiny black plastic buttons, and white stockings and shoes. "I grew up in the late sixties when drug use was popular," she continued, "but I always made a point to stay away from all that. A few years later though, I got pregnant and gave birth to my daughter. I wasn't married, and my boyfriend left me. My family didn't help at all, and I had to drop out of college to work. I was all alone and started drinking, and eventually used cocaine."

She looked down in her lap sadly, then took a deep breath. "A coworker saw in me what I didn't know was happening to myself. He sat and talked to me, and I broke down and cried. He asked me if I wanted to go away to get help, and I nodded yes. My workplace and union made all the necessary arrangements, and that's how I ended up at a rehab in Weston, Georgia.

"There I had a physical exam. They mentioned they were testing for HIV. But since I wasn't an intravenous drug user and I thought all my sexual partners were okay, I wasn't afraid at all. I had seen information about AIDS, and I knew about GMHC [the Gay Men's Health Crisis, an organization in New York City founded to help people with AIDS]. But I had never read the fine print. I thought of HIV/AIDS as basically a gay issue.

"At the rehab there was a young lady who was HIV positive, and I 'judged' her. She asked to borrow my lipstick, and I let her. But when she returned it, I told her she could keep it. I knew I was never going to use it again, now that she had.

"Two weeks later the counselor called me into his office. There was the director of the program and also this same young lady. They told me that the lab results came back and that I had tested positive. The girl who was positive hugged me, and the counselor hugged me, and I sat there in a state of total shock. I was frightened, but I didn't even know what of. I just sat there. I couldn't even respond when they asked me questions. Then, suddenly, I just started screaming at the top of my lungs and sobbing uncontrollably. I was totally lost.

"I called home and told my family, and they said, 'It isn't true. It isn't possible. You're in Georgia: they don't know what they're talking about.' That's what I wanted to believe too, so I did.

"But when I refused to believe the results, the rehab ordered a second test. It came back positive too. I asked to see the sheet of paper with the results printed on it in black and white, and I still have that piece of paper today.

"The rehab also wanted me to call and tell all my sexual partners from the previous five years. So I had to make a list, and it was then I felt the impact of where the drinking and cocaine had taken me, because it was a very long list. In this rehab I had seen some young ladies who had been on a roll, selling their bodies to support their habit, and I had always had this better-than-you attitude because I had never done that. But then the shame hit me that no, I had done it for free. I was scheduled to see a psychiatrist at the rehab, but I never went. He said that if I didn't open up and talk to him, he couldn't help me. But at that point I just didn't give a damn.

"When I left, the rehab suggested that I attend an AA meeting back here in New York and tell people about my addiction. But they told me not to mention my HIV status because I might face prejudice and rejection that I wouldn't be ready to handle. So I had this secret. I went to a meeting, and just said, 'This is my first time here,' and everybody hugged me. It was a real warm feeling, so I just put the HIV issue aside: 'No, it's just nonexistent.'

"Eventually I thought I was okay with the diagnosis. But I had to be retested here in New York. While waiting for the results I kept hoping they had made a mistake in Georgia—that they had switched my blood with that other girl's. I held on to that glimmer of hope. But the results came back the same.

"I wanted everything to go on as normal. I had never been on public assistance and didn't want to start now, so I kept my job. This was my way of being a normal member of society and not clumped with HIV-AIDS kinds of things.

"Still, periodically, clouds of despair come over me. I feel ugly— a freak. I just keep thinking that before HIV I was fine. I also have sometimes thought HIV was my payment for promiscuity. I thought of God as a punishing God.

"But I'm learning to talk about what I feel, no matter how ridiculous—so my ears can hear what my mouth has to say. And hopefully these feelings do pass. Now I think I'm at a point where I'm 'HIV Wilma.' When I felt like an 'HIV person' over here and just 'Wilma' over there, things clashed, because what Wilma wanted to do, HIV couldn't or wouldn't, and what HIV wanted, Wilma couldn't or wouldn't do. I would want to have sex without using a condom, but I couldn't, so it was hard for me to come together and feel this is me—'HIV Wilma,' the whole.

"Now, I don't feel I deserve HIV. It's just fate. This is what happened, and I'm who it happened to. I have choices today, and I choose to go in the right direction.

"I look at life totally differently now. This is it, this lifetime here. Nobody promised me another life, so I have to do the best I can with this one, HIV and all."

For Wilma and many others, the first intimation of illness—the result of a medical test without a corresponding change in health status—triggers disbelief. This sudden event can occur in the absence of any other experiential evidence. Wilma encountered problems in part because HIV positivity itself is not even an illness but merely the result of a test; nonetheless it turned her into a patient in her own and others' eyes. She then had to struggle to figure out what this "state" or "condition," with all its uncertainties, meant. To her, HIV connoted death, taintedness, and sin. To integrate the illness into her life and connect it with her prior view of herself posed enormous challenges. She resisted, and continued to struggle against the radical incongruity between past and present.

Even those who expect to be positive are unprepared for the shock. Jenny Singer, for example, a thirty-eight-year-old Italian-American nurse, had used intravenous drugs for several months but had stopped ten years ago and completed school. "I remember

the exact day I tested positive," she told me. "October 21, 1989—
a special day. I didn't believe the test counselor when she told me,
and I grabbed the paper out of her hand, saying, 'Let me see that.'
'All right,' she said, 'if you want to see it, here.' There were three
boxes that read: negative, retest, and positive. The last one was
checked. I had to see to make sure she wasn't making a mistake—
even though I had the feeling for a while that I was positive. I had
traveled to Mexico the year before and my husband and I had
both gotten salmonella. He recovered in a week, and it took me
four months! Yet I still didn't expect the test to be positive because
I'd been healthy ever since I had given up drugs ten years before.
When she told me, I was shocked. I felt like one of those big Chi-
nese gongs that gets hit with a hammer. Everything was vibrating.
I didn't hear whatever else she said. I remember it was raining outside and I went afterward with my husband to a diner to have a
cup of coffee. He went to the bathroom and I sat around looking
at all these people, feeling totally out of place . . . a leper." The
world now seemed different to her. She had lost her sense of fitting
in.

Such initial reactions can be delayed. Reynaldo Fernandez, a
hefty, muscular, thirty-three-year-old heterosexual Latino with a
history of injecting drug use, had a shaved head and wore large
glasses with thick black plastic frames, the lenses magnifying his
eyes. "It didn't hit me that bad or heavy, sitting inside the counselor's office," he reported. "She explained it to me, and I said,
'Yeah, I know all the data and everything.' Not until I went outside did it hit. I wanted to find a hole to crawl in. I almost walked
into a couple of trees and poles without thinking, and crossed the
street without looking. The first thing I did was go to buy a watch.
I had needed one for a while, but I finally went and bought one.
Then I stood in a phone booth and called my girlfriend. But it still
didn't feel real. It wasn't until a few weeks later that I began to
deal with it."

As a result of these discontinuities, many avoid getting tested in the first place. Yvette Bing, a forty-two-year-old African-American woman with a history of drug use, said, "Before getting tested, I talked to people who had been diagnosed. They confirmed what I felt: don't be tested. Ignorance is bliss. It's better not to know. I got tested five times because my drug programs made me, but I never went to pick up the results. Each day is easier to contend with if I have 'forever' to live."

Markers

The course of change for these patients is not smooth but step-wise. A series of chapters unfolds, each representing loss. Through this process, who one is—one's sense of self—is transformed. Many view these experiences of infection as a journey—a concept that can organize and frame events. Voyages, after all, have desti-nations and stages. The unexpected, in retrospect, becomes seen as logical outcome.

Many infected individuals don't feel anything is wrong until their T-cells or CD-4 counts begin to fall.* As Todd Crenshaw, a twenty-nine-year-old gay man who had been studying to be a physician's assistant, told me, "I thought I was fine until my T-cells dropped. That's when I realized that yes, indeed, something was the matter with me. Before then I hadn't paid much attention to the fact I was positive. It didn't bother me. I didn't think about it."

For others the development of physical symptoms marks the first critical transition. Roy Gifford, a forty-nine-year-old gay man

---

*T-cells, a variety of lymphocytes or white blood cells, consist of two sub-types: T4 (or helper) cells that HIV attacks, and T8 (or suppressor) cells. Pa-tients referring to "T-cells" usually mean T4 cells or the ratio of T4 to T8 cells. T4 cells are so named because of the presence on them of CD4 recep-tors. Hence blood tests for T4 cells are also known as "CD4 counts."

about to retire because of HIV, said, "Until recently, I took nasty little pills every four hours—a total of sixty-five a day—but didn't consider myself sick. Then suddenly one day at work I felt drained. I realized then that things weren't as I had thought."

Yet, as Roy points out, he and others must decide whether to define themselves as ill. They enter a nebulous terrain due in part to the protean nature of the disease. "HIV is different in everyone," he explained, "and therefore a unique experience. This disease is not like a common cold that goes from A to B to C: first congestion, then a cough, etc., etc. New things pop up all the time: lymphomas, and mysterious things they can't even diagnose." He had been able to dismiss earlier symptoms as unrelated to the virus *per se*. There is room for him and others to interpret events in different ways.

For some patients the development of visible, as opposed to felt but invisible, symptoms marks the major turning point. Wilma says, "I gradually began to accept the diagnosis, but then I started to lose weight. I had to hide it by wearing extra clothes. I would put on three pairs of pants, or two pairs and cable tights—even in summer. I also had to change my makeup and got very upset all over again. There's an 'AIDS look' that I wanted to avoid at all costs. I didn't want to walk down the street and have everybody know. When you 'look it,' it's no longer your choice.

"Then I got my first symptoms of fatigue. I wondered, Is this 'it'? The beginning of the end? Will it all be downhill from now on? At each of these points I had to accept it all over again, as if newly diagnosed, and decide how to deal with it, whether to tell people."

For others the development of visible and specifically AIDS-diagnostic symptoms marks the critical stage. Kerry Musgrove, a forty-two-year-old gay man, now works for an HIV services organization. "I went on vacation to Puerto Rico with a friend who has AIDS," he told me. "We got to the beach in San Juan and he said, 'I think we should talk about those marks on your back.' I said, 'What marks?' I hadn't been tested and didn't know my HIV status. I was on the beach for about fifteen minutes, turned around, and flew home. Even though most of the lesions are gone or under control now, I haven't been on a beach since and won't take my clothes off again in public. A skin lesion is a literal stigma." According to the Oxford English Dictionary, the word *stigma* itself derives from Greek, referring to "a mark made on the skin by pricking, cutting or branding." Later the term came to refer to "marks resembling the wounds on Jesus' crucified body," and "a mark or sign of disgrace or discredit." Visible symptoms take on significance because of their social as well as medical implications.

Symptoms—even if they are still invisible—that meet the diagnostic criteria for AIDS, as opposed to HIV infection alone, can nonetheless change one's sense of self. Maurice Bradford, a forty-four-year-old gay man, had been a successful health care administrator. He met me in my office and was neatly groomed with short-cut light brown hair. He wore a jacket and tie. "Some people have been HIV-positive for years and never gotten sick," he said. "It wasn't until I got PCP"—pneumocystis carinii pneumonia, an opportunistic infection that is an indicator of AIDS— "that I thought, 'Oh, fuck, this is for real. This is HIV.' Up to that point all I had was rotten lab work. I had gotten tested only as a precautionary step, never thinking I'd be positive. I had thought there would have been some sign before then. But there wasn't.

"So when I got pneumonia and had to be hospitalized, I realized I would not be one of the lucky ones. I still can't believe it." He shook his head. "Things like this don't happen to me. I've always been successful at whatever I tried to do." He had lost his sense of himself as moving smoothly ahead in life. Even for gay men, heavily affected as a group by the epidemic, HIV is outside the range of normal expectable events.

Eventually Maurice recovered from PCP and returned to work, but the following year he developed shingles. Such medical crises, interspersed with periods of relative good health, "feel like a roller coaster." Symptoms and the emotional upheaval they bring come and go and with them a flip-flopping between crisis and normalcy, life and death.

For some, the point at which they need medications marks the major turning point. Alfie Montoya, a forty-six-year-old Latino who had been an injecting drug user, "had been diagnosed for a couple of years. But when I went to the pharmacy and got AZT, I looked at the pills in my hand and said, 'Man!' I cried. I still wanted to believe they had made a mistake with the diagnosis, that I wasn't actually infected—even though I had had shingles. When I needed to take the medicine, I saw that I really had this shit." Again, these events break through denial, numbness, and the desire to continue life as it is. Alfie and others are then forced against their will to incorporate the possibility of death into their lives.

One-way Streets: Losses

Clearly the potential loss of one's own life looms ultimately, yet other losses intimate and prefigure it. Medical events acquire psychological and social meanings. They represent threats to independence and functioning that can prove far more upsetting than the events themselves. "I'm on a one-way street, headed south," Aaron Eliot, a fifty-seven-year-old gay man, told me one afternoon in his small one-bedroom apartment on the Upper West Side of Manhattan. "For three and a half years I had gravy—was fine with no problems. Then the shit hit the fan. I had crypto, an inflamed gallbladder, and fevers.

"The quality of my life now is horrible. I go out once every other day, buy a newspaper, drag my groceries home, and don't go out again unless to a doctor. That's my life at this point. That's the size of it.

"Sometimes I sit in my apartment immobilized. I can't get up at all. I wait until the last possible minute to go to the bathroom or to eat, take a pill, brush my teeth or shave. I'll say, 'I'll do it in a half-hour.' I just lie here and say, 'I have to do this, I have to do that, take care of bills, get out checks.' I was always a type A personality. If I received a bill, the next day I sent it out. I always tried to do everything on time. I still try, but the pain is too much. I say, 'What for?' The end of the road is coming. I know.

"I have medications here all over the place. I come home with three, four, five, prescriptions. I'm a walking drugstore but still in limbo. Sometimes I say, 'Aaron, you're still walking!' I can't believe it. I'm still functioning—not as a full person, but minimally. I can take care of myself and get around if I have to. I figured I'd be dead now, that something would hit me, a brain infection, meningitis, or CMV retinitis [a retinal infection which can cause blindness].

"When I first got sick, my sister in Florida said to me, 'Don't expect us to hold your hand.' I'll never forget that. I'd been very close to my family, my two sisters. But if I got sick, there'd be no one there to take care of me.

"I'd been independent ever since I got out of the army. I never moved back home because I wanted my privacy. But that makes it harder now.

"My life is horrible. It's just going on and on, and it's only going to get worse. I know that. It's futile. This disease is torturous, a nightmare's nightmare, a never-ending story. It's like we're living in a third world country.

"I don't want a slow death, but it's going to happen, as it has to everybody else. A slow, horrible death. I'll be lucky if I walk down the street and have a heart attack. That would be a blessing at this point. I don't fear dying, only being sick for a long time beforehand, uncomfortable and distressed." These declines in functioning are difficult for Aaron because he sees them as stops along a "one-way highway," foreshadowing an eventual loss of life. For him, the disease represents progressive loss.

Dis-in-te-grate

For others, HIV is disturbing chiefly because of potential degradation of the mind, of a coherent self that can control the body. Olana Ramirez, a thirty-two-year-old Latina woman, arrived to meet me wearing a red jacket, a yellow shirt, blue glass teardrop earrings, purple eye shadow, and eyeliner. She had a round face and long full light brown hair that swayed as she spoke. "I am most afraid of neurological problems," she told me. "The virus entering my central nervous system indicates a real finality. I don't want to go brain dead and still walk around, or be hooked up to a machine, dying little by little. Sometimes I get numbness and don't hold my bladder the way I should—my signals are not right. They're planning to give me a CAT scan to see what's going on, which scares me. I feel I have dealt very well with this virus for many years. PCP, TB—you name it, I've dealt with it. But when it comes to the brain, I cannot fight, which frightens me. If I get brain damaged, I'd lose my thoughts—everything. What would I do? The virus will have found my weak spot. It didn't get me this way or that, so now it's trying something else. I hate this disease. I consider myself lucky because some people have it just a couple of months and then are in the hospital, losing weight, unable to walk, losing their thoughts, and not knowing where they are. I don't know how to say that word—*dis-in-te-grate*—that's spooky. When I see somebody in that state who a month or two earlier was the same as me, I have to be thankful. I'm grateful for having gotten through these other stages. If I were to see that end coming, I've contemplated taking pills."

Lost Dreams

HIV can also lead to a significant collapse of social and economic status, current or future. Todd Crenshaw, who had been studying to be a physician's assistant, said, "My status has changed completely since I've become HIV-positive." He is short with dark brown hair and a crew cut, and wore a white T-shirt, a black leather jacket, and black sneakers. "My identity's been stripped away from me," he continued. "Society has pushed me into a category. I have to associate with people with whom I normally wouldn't, simply because I have a disease I didn't ask for. I'm living on friends' couches—homeless but with a roof over my head. Until I became infected I was very much white middle-class America. That's how I was brought up. I didn't associate with drug dealers or users. I don't like being around them, having to fear for my wallet or coat. When I volunteered at GMHC as a buddy, the first thing my initial client—an IVDU—told me was 'Never trust an addict. They'll do anything for a fix.' That always stuck in my mind. Now AIDS has become my identity, which is hard since I really never had anything else to hold onto, like 'this is what Todd is.'

"There's no way I'm going to become a productive member of society again. I had been independent for years, and now I'm very dependent on others. I basically can't take care of myself. And it's only going to get worse. I don't have the energy to work full-time, but if I work part-time I jeopardize my benefits and insurance.

Two weeks in the hospital already cost me $20,000. I had private insurance and a private doctor, and the medical bills from my first hospitalization wiped out all my money. Now I'm broke. A friend of mine who's also HIV positive said he only had a year to live, and he charged all his cards to the limit and exceeded it. He gambled and traveled over the world. But when he was supposed to die, he was still alive and healthy."

Many mourn the loss of their future. Roy Gifford, for example, about to retire, said, "I had frugally saved money for years. In high school I worked three jobs, played the stock market, collected and stored away antiques, and was then able to put myself through college. I wanted to do certain things in life—like travel—that I knew would require money. I expected to have at least one, possibly two Ph.D.'s by now. I had the areas already laid out. As an undergraduate I delivered papers at Harvard. At one time I was rather brilliant. But I've just thrown out the notes I was going to base my master's work on. They were one more thing cluttering my life, one more unfulfilled dream.

"I can't plan for a future now. What's the point of thinking about tomorrow when tomorrow—or even next week—may not come? What's the point of worrying about retirement funds when I probably won't be around? I'm rather fatalistic. Too many times plans have fallen through. The old line is accurate: birth and death are the only two certainties. Everything between them is filler. I can run as much as I want, but my tail will always catch up with me.

"I wanted a small house with fruit trees and animals, and a relationship. Not 2.1 children, but freedom. I've had to forget those dreams and let them fade into the past." This loss of dreams powerfully disturbs him.

The future constitutes an important part of one's life and raison d'être. Although we can't predict the future, we make assumptions about it. Maurice Bradford, the health care administrator, said that when he tested positive, "I was about to leave my current job and start something new, and was looking forward to the prospect of moving on. I had killed myself working and going to business school full-time for a year and a half, doing reasonably well, and making contacts I thought would be helpful. Now, suddenly, that wasn't going to be practical. These implications of my HIV status, as much as being HIV positive itself, upset me. I had been oriented toward long-term planning way into the future, and working today at something as a foundation for tomorrow. Now I can't look forward to a long career, or any career. I have not been able even to consider a relationship. I don't know how much time I have." The future has been ripped away; the past no longer makes sense. Patients feel they live in a foreshortened present of unknown duration. Stability, taken for granted until now, disappears.

Lost Lives

In an epidemic, the loss of others foreshadows the possible eventual loss of self. Social and public events blur with inner experience. As Aaron Eliot, who felt he was on a "one-way street," said, "A friend of mine with the virus wasted away into a living skeleton, sunk in, barely aware of me. He sat drooling, and at one point threw up all over me. I got up and kissed him goodbye and said I'd see him next week. But the next week I was busy. The week after that his mother called and said he had gone into a coma and passed away. I'd seen pictures on TV, but it's different seeing a friend die, knowing how he looked before. He was the first person I really watched deteriorate one-on-one."

As Reynaldo Fernandez, who initially delayed his reaction, said, "Everybody I used to get high with is dead now. I'm the only one still alive of the whole crowd, and that scares the hell out of me. I had a dream I was walking through an AIDS ward looking at the patients. All of a sudden I was not walking but being taken in there on a stretcher. I woke up in sweats." He suggests a transition, a transfer between other patients and himself. He sees their fate in his, and vice versa.

The virus's transmissibility links one to the potential death of others even more. As Todd Crenshaw said, "I feel like I'm a walking time bomb." Although stable for the moment, he feels dangerous, threatening to destroy himself and people around him with both contagion and rage.

These losses merge over time—reminders of mortality. Painful, even if anticipated, their import cannot be fully imagined until experienced. The losses and stresses accumulate and combine. As Maurice Bradford explained, "I spent the first week after testing grieving the loss of my relationship and of future work prospects, arranging for my own health needs, planning to make sure I had enough insurance and income, getting used to seeing my future as a lot bleaker than it had been, and dealing with the death of two friends who had died that very same week. It's hard to separate my HIV status from these other things—particularly my lover suddenly dumping me, which hurt more than testing positive itself."

HIV infection constitutes a journey for infected individuals, who experience it in different ways. The point at which they first begin to confront the infection varies, and disbelief, alienation, and delay commonly occur. A long series of events follows, including lab tests and symptoms—visible and unseen, specific to HIV, diagnostic of AIDS, and requiring medication. A series of losses also ensues—of function, mind, future, socioeconomic status, and friends. These transitions and stresses produce a roller-coaster effect as individuals struggle to find ways to cope.

TWO

Taboos

PROBLEMS EMERGE due not only to losses but to stigma, which complicates the course of HIV. The illness affects patients' views of themselves in their own and others' eyes. The infected come to feel "taboo" and like "second-class citizens." Discrimination arises from families, communities, health care workers, and work settings, and varies in form, content, and social and psychological import.

Paper Plates: Rejection from Families

For Lorraina Ortiz, a thirty-two-year-old Latina, "The hardest part of having HIV is rejection, being labeled. In the hospital I told my mother in tears that the doctor had said I had AIDS. My mother looked at me, didn't say anything, and just walked out. I didn't see her again for two years. She's an educated woman, but at that time HIV equaled AIDS, and she treated me as if I were a leper. That was the worst rejection I faced, right there. I called her and went to her house, but she refused to see me. Either she wouldn't answer the door, or somebody else would answer and say she wasn't there, and I wasn't allowed in because she was out. Once, I knew she was home because her car was outside, but she sent out a girl who takes care of her to say, 'Your mother's not here. Next time call before you come. She doesn't want you around the neighborhood.' But when I called, my mother was always going out, or was too busy and had no time. She'd say, 'Call me next week.' But when I called, she'd have her answering machine on. I never got to talk to her. After a while, she said, 'Look, don't call me. I'm not ready to talk to you. You should have thought about this before you did what you did. This happened to you because you wanted it. Now you have to deal with it. What am I going to tell people? That my daughter has AIDS?'

"As a woman, I needed my mother to talk to. She's the only person I really have. I have brothers, but no sisters.

"After two years, my son wanted to see me. He was fourteen and was living with my mother at the time. He called me and said, 'I want to see you. Meet me at the shopping center near grandma's house on Tuesday.'

"I used to speak with him and tell him, 'I need to talk to grandma. I'm going through a lot.' And he would say, 'Yeah, I know what's going on. But grandma doesn't want to see you. She's hurting.'

"So he planned to meet me. But as I walked across to him, I saw my mother standing there with him, holding packages. She didn't know I was going to be there, and suddenly we were face to face. I said, 'Mom, I really want to talk to you,' and we just stood there. I could tell that she wanted to cry. Finally, she said, 'Okay, let's go to the house.' So we went and sat down. She said she was going through a lot because she couldn't accept that I was an addict. She had brought me up a certain way and I turned out to be the opposite. How could she tell people about my HIV status?" Lorraina had other relatives with substance abuse problems. But that did not alleviate her mother's anger and rejection. Her mother had all the more hoped that Lorraina would not fall prey to the same fate.

"Since then," Lorraina continued, "I talk to her, but she still hasn't really accepted me. She lets me go to her house once a year. I call her, but she won't call me. I try to phone her twice, sometimes three times a week, depending on how long she lets me stay on the phone. When we do talk, it's very depressing because she brings up my past and condemns me a lot. It's not a supportive mother-daughter relationship. Sometimes I wonder why I'm wasting my time, hearing reminders of how I got it. Everything she says is negative. She's punishing me.

"When I visit her, I can't eat from her plates or drink from the same cups. She sets the table with real plates and cups for everyone else, and paper plates, a paper cup, and plastic silverware for me.

"She also told my father, which I didn't feel she had a right to do. It was up to me. I can't talk to him now like I used to. I feel he's judging me. He doesn't want to hear about it. When it comes up, he changes the subject or walks out of the room. He doesn't let me tell him, 'Daddy, it happened. It's something we can't go back on. The harm is already done.' To him, the lowest thing is that I was a drug addict and a prostitute. Now he doesn't want to be bothered with me at all.

"One of my greatest fears is ending up in the hospital. I'm not scared of dying but of the process of getting sick, and deteriorating, finding myself helpless in bed, because I wouldn't want my mother to go through it. When I was twenty-four years old, using drugs, I did a lot of shit out there to her and to my family, and I wouldn't want her to see me just ending up helpless, a burden to care for.

"Some people who know I'm HIV stay away from me because they're afraid they might catch it, and they think they're better than me. It makes me feel guilty about things I did in the past. I think, 'There go the healthy people, and there go the sick.' Two girls I know were kicked out of their house by their own mother. Even people in the AIDS field tend to look at me like I'm on the doomsday line."

Gay men, too, often faced rejection from their families, even before HIV. Some families reject homosexuality because of church teachings. As Todd Crenshaw, who had complained about his loss of socioeconomic status, explained, "In my family it's still taboo to talk about homosexuality. If anybody knows, they don't say anything. They feel it's against God's will for two men to be together."

Many gay men face difficulties from their lovers' families as well. Maurice Bradford, the health care administrator, says, "I am the primary executor of my former companion's estate. His evil bitch sister in Chicago has challenged the will, thinking she was going to get wealthy. I've had to spend the little money left in the estate on lawyers. For the last year and a half of his life, I took care of him—everything from feeding to nursing him. I not only took care of him but put up with him. At times he was horrible— hostile and bitter beyond belief, noncommunicative, uncooperative, refusing to take care of himself or take his medicine, and being very unsupportive of me, though I was also positive. She never visited him when he was sick or gave a shit about him. I can't understand why she is now doing this. It's more than just greed, it's viciousness. She's trying to hurt me. She's self-righteous and stubborn, pursuing this case to the very end. A jury trial starts next month. I just keep thinking: what the fuck did I do wrong?" As with many gay men, Maurice is tempted to blame himself as a result of the widespread rejection he has encountered since growing up.

Walk-ups: Rejection from Communities

Stigma also arises from communities, both gay and straight. As Todd Crenshaw explained, "Even in the gay community and the HIV-positive community there is a lot of stigma. I went to a Body Positive social for HIV-positive people. It was in a fourth-floor walk-up, and it was almost impossible for those of us with AIDS fatigue to get up the stairs. Once I got there it was like a gay bar. Everyone was standing and modeling, which I never was really into anyway. Everybody also denied having ARC [AIDS Related Complex, a diagnosis formerly used to describe a condition between HIV infection without symptoms and full-blown AIDS] or AIDS, and said they were just HIV positive—even those I had had dinner with at GMHC, where you have to have AIDS to get in. In the gay community there are 'positives' and 'negatives.' " He separated the two with his hands in the air. "When I've met and told some people I'm positive, a mist comes down in front of their face. I had a date with a guy I met in the gym who had expressed a lot of interest in me. But when I said I was positive, the date just ended right there. He never called me again."

Within the gay community, positives often keep their own company, with separation imposed by both themselves and others. Todd Crenshaw explained, "I prefer to spend my time with other people who are positive. They're the only ones who can really understand what I'm going through. As a lot more gay men are getting tested, the polarization of negatives and positives is becoming stronger. I sense a separation: people who are negative are pure, clean, and okay, and the rest of us are tainted. I really began to feel it strongly about two years ago. Before that I hardly experienced it at all. Nobody ever asked me my status or brought it up. I get angry at people labeling me based on it. I met a guy at a bus stop who sat down next to me, and began cruising me, trying to pick me up. Within the first ten minutes he managed to tell me he was HIV negative and asked if I had been tested. I thought, what the fuck are you doing? How dare you ask me a personal question like that, and why the hell would it matter? If I tell you I'm negative, is that going to affect what you do with me sexually? Because if it does, you're an idiot. I could lie, or could have been negative six months ago and be positive now. It's worthless information." His reasoning is legitimate. Yet he debases the information in part because it has also had painful repercussions for him.

Several gay men were abandoned by their lovers after testing positively. Maurice Bradford added, "Within a week of testing, the person I was involved with ended the relationship. He fantasized and fabricated horrible reasons for my being unworthy of a relationship, and basically threw me out. He didn't say, 'I can't deal with you because you're HIV positive.' He came up with all kinds of crazy things. His friends were shocked. They didn't understand. I knew what it was: he was throwing me and my HIV infection out at the same time. That's what made it devastating."

Segregation occurs within other communities as well. "If people on my parents' block found out," Jill Montgomery, an African-American woman who grew up in the inner city, reported, "my parents would be ostracized by their neighbors." Often segregation arises from unexpected sources. Jenny Singer, who had worked as a nurse, described how an AIDS services organization offered "scattered-site housing," arranging for her to have an apartment, but "recommended that I don't tell my neighbors that I'm HIV positive, or let anybody know my business since it could lead to problems. They told me to keep it to myself. I feel kind of bad. I don't get involved in anything. I've been there for six months, and nobody on the block knows me." The agency's recommendation inadvertently added to her own sense of being diseased. "Our next-door neighbor doesn't talk to us. The back of the building has just two apartments—theirs and ours. But our neighbors knew that the people there before us had AIDS. So the neighbors probably know that we do too. Every night they spray disinfectant in the hall. Then Carl, my boyfriend, goes out and sprays *his* disinfectant, just to get back at them. When they see us, they walk the other way."

Three Gloves: Rejection from Health Care Workers

Health care workers and institutions shape patients' approaches toward HIV, but they also stigmatize patients. That, Wilma Smith says, "hurts the most. They of all people should know better. One x-ray technician, as soon as he saw 'HIV' in my chart, put on two masks, two gowns, and three pairs of gloves. He took one x-ray film and then had to do another. So he helped me onto the table—with two gloves on—and then took those off and put on two other pairs. It upset me. Aren't these people informed? The guy didn't even realize how silly he looked. Also in my clinic, my chart is plastered with a big red sticker, meaning I am HIV. In this clinic they give us patients our charts to carry around to the specialty clinics. So I had to lug the chart around with this big red sticker. It doesn't say 'HIV' on it, but everyone knows what it is, and the staff all look at me kind of funny. Even the receptionists at the desk look at me as if to say, 'I know what you got, honey.' "

Gerry Galvez, a thirty-eight-year-old Latina woman and former injecting drug user, told me, "When I was in the hospital two years ago, an orderly used to come in to clean my room, and he always talked to me. He'd bring me flowers left by other patients, or cake from the kitchen. He knew I liked cake. He'd come on his breaks too.

"Then the nurse put one of those big Infectious Disease signs on the outside of my door, saying that visitors had to scrub and put on all this garbage, and he stopped coming. The food workers wouldn't even bring my meals into the room anymore. They just left them in front of the door, afraid they would catch something by walking in. Even in my clinic, when I try to give the nurses the little tube with the urine specimen in it, I ask, 'What do you want me to do with this?' Sometimes they just grab it out of my hand and put it in the container, but some of them say, 'Put it in that box, right over there. I'm not touching it.' I feel as if just talking to me is going to give it to them, like my whole being is just one big infectious disease.

"It's also difficult to take my blood sometimes because I'm an ex-IV drug user. One nurse was jabbing and sticking me. I always try to hold on and think it will be over soon. But she wanted to go into my leg. I told her no. She got pissed off because blood was all over the place. She walked out with gobs of protective stuff on and said something about 'that AIDS patient!' But you can't tell me I have AIDS because I don't. I'm only HIV. So when she came back in, I was crying. I was trying to follow what they say in AA: 'Let go and let God,' and 'If it doesn't apply, let it fly.' But it just wasn't working."

Hidden Bottles: Rejection at Work

Stigma arises in professional as well as personal contexts. Fears of job loss perpetuate secrecy. This problem particularly plagues HIV-infected health care workers, who face added burdens because of public fear they might transmit the virus to their patients.

Public discourse on health care workers and HIV changed as a result of Kimberly Bergalis allegedly becoming infected by her Florida dentist, Dr. David Acer. Before, it was the possibility of physicians, blood drawers, and other health care workers contracting HIV from patients that had received press attention. Now physicians and other health care workers themselves are

seen as possible sources of contagion. They are distrusted—
though Dr. Acer has remained the only health care worker with
purported evidence of having infected any patients. This switch
owes much to implicit homophobia and moral revulsion toward
those with HIV.

"I lead a double life," Jenny Singer, the nurse, said, "as if I were
a split personality. People are always telling me, 'Oh, you're a
nurse, an intelligent girl, you should have known better.' But it's
not intelligence, it's an emotional problem. I had low self-esteem,
having been physically abused by my father, and had used drugs a
few times. I gave them up ten years ago and went to nursing
school, but I can never escape my past. It seems unfair to have
worked so hard to get clean and then find out I have the virus. I'm
mad at myself. I've seen a lot of friends die from it. So many young
people get sick and die after they have straightened out their lives
and gotten back on the right track. They're being punished all
their lives for a mistake they made. My drug addiction is a weight
I can never get rid of. I got my life together, but I'm still stuck with
this thing, and it keeps coming back in my face, following me
around. It's always going to be there, held against me. If I were
Betty Ford and had a lot of money, I'd be a hero. That's how it
works. But I don't understand why I'm always paying for it; I really don't. I don't think God punishes people like this. But I can't
find an explanation.

"My coworkers' attitudes outrage me. Well-educated nurses and
doctors say, 'I'd never take care of a person with AIDS because
everything isn't known about it, and I wouldn't risk my life. I have
to think of my children. People with the virus deserve it. Look at
the kind of life they're living.'

"Sitting around, one secretary said, 'When I go to church I'm
afraid to drink from the cup because somebody with AIDS might
have drank from it.' Then another woman I work with said, 'Oh,
you don't have to worry about that. Those type of people don't go

to church.' I listen to stuff like that and feel very out of place. We screened patients for the nursing home, and if they had AIDS the medical director would say, 'I don't want these goddamn pieces of shit with AIDS in our facility.'

"So I was very concerned that anyone would know I had it because I might lose my license and my job. I didn't tell anybody. I had to hide that I had used drugs and had HIV. I've always had to hide something and felt people were going to find out something about me. At work I was one way, and at home another. I always had to lie. I felt like two different people.

"A section of me lived here, a section there. Only part, not all of me would be at work. I appeared there in fragments at times. I finally told one coworker but made her promise not to tell anyone else. That's the worst part of HIV: having to hide it. When I had to take my medication, I pretended to be going to the bathroom and carried my purse with me. I kept my medications in a little Tylenol bottle in case someone saw. It was stressful. Rumors went around that I was using crack because I had lost close to twenty-five pounds and was so skinny and out sick so much.

"The people I worked with had liked me very much. I wish that before I left I had said, 'You like me, but I have AIDS. Maybe your thoughts about the disease are wrong.'"

Health care workers also see the devastation wreaked by the virus on patients. "When I think about HIV," Jenny reflected, "I think about a woman in a coma at a nursing home in Brooklyn where I worked. She had big bed sores all over her body. One had eaten away her ear. I turned her over every half-hour. When I think 'HIV' today, I think about that girl and how fast the virus ate away at her." The virus's aggressiveness becomes concrete—the work of "the enemy."

Employment as a health care worker can provide insight and perspective on the illness. "When I was working in a nursing home, patients were dying all the time, and it made me more aware of my life and how I live it." But difficulties overshadow these advantages.

Stigma from work adds to that from other sources. "My side of the family has mostly been positive and supportive," Jenny continued. "But one of my aunts with four grandchildren said, 'You can still see the children as long as you don't get sick.' I have even more of a problem with my boyfriend's mother, who takes care of his three nieces. Every time we go over there, she hides them in the back bedroom and closes the door or sends them out into the street. She doesn't want us to be near them. Carl has tried to talk to her about it, but she doesn't understand or want to." This separation serves as a premonition, too, of what will occur at death.

"For a long time," Jenny confessed, "I felt like a big germ—an infected person, tainted, able to infect other people. HIV is like leprosy. Lepers were outcasts, separated from everybody else and thrown together on an island to isolate them. That's how I felt. I'm sure people like Jesse Helms would like to round us up and throw us in a camp somewhere. The government now has a ban on letting people with the virus into this country."

Those with a taboo disease become themselves taboo, defined by their disease. Their sense of isolation increases as their identity becomes restructured in others' eyes. These changes become internalized as well. Jenny and others not only feel stigmatized but come to see themselves as 'abnormal.' "I try to pretend I'm normal," she said, "even though I have HIV." Certainly the "norm"—the most common condition—is not to be infected. But to see HIV as not being normal suggests more. Many say they wish they were normal—i.e., HIV negative—in a way not found with other illnesses, reflecting widespread stigma. According to the Oxford English Dictionary, *norm* derives from the Latin word for "a carpenter's square pattern, rule." *Normal* means "right angled, constituting and conforming to a type or standard; regular, usual, typical; ordinary, conventional. Also, physically or mentally sound, healthy; heterosexual." The term thus blends the usual, the healthy, and the heterosexual and carries a moral overtone.

Many patients feel both contaminated and contaminating. As Reynaldo Fernandez, the heterosexual man who had a nightmare of being on an AIDS ward, said, "My semen is now poison." "Seed" can now both create and kill life. Thus HIV can exacerbate conceptions of the self as damaged or flawed.

Sick Roles

Many infected individuals are placed in the "sick role" and viewed as if they are about to die. First described by the sociologist Talcott Parsons, the sick role consists of exemptions from ordinary burdens, and the obligation to do everything possible to get better. Ken Landers, a thirty-one-year-old gay man who had struggled for several years trying to succeed as an actor, recently had to move back home with his suburban parents. "They treat me as if I'm china that's about to break," he told me, "as if they're walking on eggshells. My mother pampers me. I have a low platelet count. She's very leery of me doing any work, because she's afraid that if I get cut I won't stop bleeding. I keep telling her I'm a grown man, just leave me alone. I appreciate her concern, but she's overdoing it. She's too overprotective, which makes me mad. She forgets I'm thirty-one and thinks I'm still thirteen. I wash my own clothes. I have my own silverware and plates and my own place where I put them aside from my mother's. My family is overwhelming—bothering me, telling me about this new treatment or that. It makes me feel I always have to run after my life." Thus a tension exists between viewing HIV infection as acute (imminently life-threatening) or chronic—a condition one can live with for a prolonged period.

Yet without the sick role, problems emerge. Raoul Rodriquez, a thirty-two-year-old gay Mexican schoolteacher, lives with his sister in New Jersey. "My sister is generally supportive," he told me, "but sometimes I need more. Sometimes my room is a mess: I'm taking pills and have three cups there and am depressed. She comes in and says, 'C'mon, you're leaving all the cups here.' I feel like saying, 'C'mon, I have AIDS—a real problem in my life—and you're worried because three cups are here!' Sometimes I notice that she really cares and doesn't want to let me know. She gets scared, for example, if I start coughing." The sick role can thus confer advantages, legitimizing the disease so that infected persons are not blamed or seen as socially deviant. In contrast, Lorraina, for example, encounters both of these attitudes from her family, who refuse to accept or support her.

Apartheid

Issues of death and social injustice come together to trigger images of genocides that have littered twentieth-century history—the widespread killing of particular cultural groups. Many infected individuals already belong to groups that face discrimination—gay men, African Americans, and Latinos. HIV exacerbates existing feelings of social injustice, furthering the sense of social fragmentation, of "us and them."

Many sense neglect and hostility from the rest of society in the lack of better treatment. Others feel HIV in fact represents a government plot. Olana Ramirez, who feared disintegration, told me, "They had a germ-warfare experiment that went wrong, and they blamed it on faggots and dope addicts." Yvette Bing, who in the past refused to pick up her test results, argued, "It's a man-made virus that the government devised. Biological or germ warfare to get rid of the four most hated groups in society—gays, blacks, Hispanics, and drug users—a population-control experiment that got more out of hand than they thought. The government did horrible things back in the thirties and the sixties. Why not again? It was very convenient for the conservatives to come up with this virus to get rid of all these groups in one fell swoop. The government may have tried it on Africans first. Why not? The government did syphilis experiments on blacks at Tuskegee. Scientists are like gods, inventing things. Maybe they invented this too. I've also heard that the CIA put it in the water in the Belgian Congo during the uprising in 1959, and that it came from Fort Detrick, Maryland"—where, in fact, experiments in biological warfare have historically been carried out, and where one building has been sealed off for decades because of escaped anthrax. "They want to do an apartheid thing on us and separate us. That's why I refuse to enter an HIV housing complex."

The significance of these assertions lies not in their veracity or lack thereof, but in the degree of disfranchisement they suggest. These beliefs may affect how much individuals feel government and medical institutions can help with services or advice. Of note, one of the final acts of the KGB before the Soviet Union's dismemberment was to promote the rumor in Africa that HIV was a U.S. government plot. Although no evidence exists that the KGB disseminated this belief in the United States, the idea's persistence here demonstrates the degree of estrangement some already feel, further perpetuated by the epidemic.

Others view the government less severely, not as part of a conspiracy but as unhelpful and unfriendly, impersonal and neglectful, providing insufficient funds for services and research.

"They could find a cure if they really wanted," Olana insisted. "But they don't because it's big business: a lot of people are making a lot of money off of HIV. Drug companies don't want to give up large profits from AZT. How much money do you think the AZT company is making? And the ddI company? A cure would cut all that. They don't want to lose their money. That's reality, that's society: there are the poor, the middle, and the rich. The only hope I have is from HIV having attacked the rich too. But then, they can afford cures. Suppose a 'big' doctor, a specialist, finds something that works really well. He would charge $500 a visit. If I go to his office, would he take care of me? I doubt it. My mother's gynecologist on Fifth Avenue charges $75 for a visit. I once had a positive Pap smear. I told him I had Medicaid and he said, 'Sorry, I don't accept that.'

"They are too quick to throw away black, low-income families without good insurance. Instead of doctors doing everything they could to keep a person alive, it's just another case gone.

"I think they're waiting to find a cure, and the first people who will get it will be upper-class. The companies will make good money on it too. If HIV was affecting more white people who had money, they would have found a cure faster. Most people don't care about those who have AIDS."

Lorraina Ortiz, rejected by her family, echoes these feelings. "They have a cure, but only 'the elites' get it. Everything is money and greed. People are flying over to Europe and getting treated and coming back here negative—but only people who can pay for it. What are they doing over there that they're not doing here? I feel the research here is not moving so fast. Not many new things have came out, so how deep is the research?" Press reports of treatments abroad, such as those Rock Hudson flew to Paris to receive, fuel these tales. A surprising number of individuals spontaneously volunteered such stories before the recent development of expensive new protease inhibitors.

The gap between how infected individuals see themselves and how they are viewed by others produces a persistent tension. Men and women with HIV get labeled, separated, and rejected by families of origin, uninfected communities, health care workers, and employers. Individuals respond differently. Previous experiences and guilt over past behavior exacerbate discrimination; and individuals vary as to which sources of stigma are "the worst." Such condemnation from others also has several consequences, impairing self-esteem. Many patients become ghettoized or come to lead a "double life." To enter the sick role can legitimize the illness and generate social support, but it can lead to problems too, as infected individuals may perceive themselves as healthier than they are seen by others. Meanwhile, discrimination—past and current—leads many patients to view the health care system with cynicism and anger. In sum, infected men and women must find ways of dealing not only with loss but with the consequences of being outcast.

Part II: ADAPTATIONS

___

THREE

HIV-Land: *The Landscape*

LOSSES AND REJECTIONS prompt several patterns of patient response—common ways of continuing on and looking for hope.
First, many individuals enter the HIV or AIDS community or
"AIDS Movement"—a subculture of HIV groups and organizations which has developed its own customs and language. It fills
needs and desires that the rest of society has been slow to meet or
refused to consider.

HIV Junkie

George Sullivan, a large fifty-five-year-old gay man and former
Wall Street executive, came to my office wearing a plaid Brooks
Brothers shirt, corduroy pants, and Topsiders. He spoke in a firm,
crisp voice. "Over the years I've become an HIV junkie," he explained. "I've read everything about the disease I could. People
have told me I should get a job in the AIDS world. My sister recently said, 'They're setting up a new AIDS Unit in New London,
Connecticut,' near her house. 'Why don't you apply for a job?' I

said, 'New London, Connecticut—what, are you kidding?' But seriously, HIV has become my whole life.

"I have a Harvard education and used to go to work in a suit, carrying a briefcase and flying to meetings around the country. Then I got the virus. I went though various self-improvement and transformation games like the Forum, to raise my self-esteem and not feel like a second-class citizen. But I felt outside the financial world where I worked. All those people were straight and HIV negative. It was very difficult to get along there as an openly gay— never mind HIV-positive—man. I just can't compete with them, with first-class citizens—straight and uninfected.

"I don't feel that way about uninfected gays. They're not that much ahead, and I try not to feel severely inferior to them. In fact, being positive has some benefits. People ask, 'Why? Are you crazy?' And I say, 'If I were negative, I'd be at much more risk of becoming positive, which could really upset me. Some people die in months after becoming infected. As I'm already positive, I only face the risk of becoming more positive from another strain of virus, and I know that my body has already been able to tolerate this infection for at least some time. So I pity those poor negatives because they're like those plastic-bubble babies—fragile and vulnerable to everything.' Some people say to me, 'Oh bullshit! I'd give my ass to be negative.' But that's how I feel.

"Sometimes we laugh that negatives are getting an inferiority complex and forming their own support groups. At first I said, 'Oh, that's so Californian.' But they feel left out because the HIV positives have all this attention and support through GMHC and groups like Body Positive. The negatives are getting neglected." Indeed, HIV-negative support groups are now sponsored by many such organizations.

Yet membership has a high cost. HIV-land is a culture of death as well as of renewal. "My whole generation in New York is dead," George continued. "All the people I knew in my age bracket are gone except for Dave who is a PWA [person with AIDS] and has only forty T-cells left. I had twenty-five close friends and fifty acquaintances die, and I stopped counting. Now those figures have doubled, and I refuse to go back and list them. It's too painful. I see their faces sometimes. I see people in a crowd and say, 'It's Jim' or 'It's Tom.' But it isn't. And I have dreams about them too.

"Occasionally some guy will come up to me on the street whom I haven't seen for years, and we'll have an unspoken ritual of saying 'Good to see you!' which means 'Glad you're alive. I didn't know. I haven't seen you and assumed you were dead.' We are few and far between, us old healthy dinosaurs, the few of us left in the community. So I live in a group, in an area which is heavily affected—heavily positive. That's HIV-land. I try to construct a new AIDS universe in which there's some security and safety, until something comes to poke a hole in it."

To manage the stresses of HIV, George and others have created their own "New World." Individuals journey into a new realm— geographically, socially, and psychologically. HIV, threatening both the individual and his world, provokes an all-encompassing response as seen with no other disease in the West today.

The ranks of HIV-land, continually diminished with death, simultaneously swell with those newly infected. Many enter, yet none can fully leave. Some may drift out but remain marked as members. The boundary with the outside world is demarcated, tense, and truly permeable in only one direction.

Yet HIV-land has helped George and others in innumerable ways. This "New AIDS Universe" provides a new cosmology, in the sense of the Greek word cosmos, meaning both "world" and "order." At the center of HIV-land, groups and organizations of the infected seek order and wholeness in the midst of biological, psychological, social, and economic devastation. As one world crumbles, a new one is born.

The HIV community provides George and others with tangible benefits, including legal assistance, advice in negotiating with physicians and the medical system, and free meals and clothing; and it performs numerous psychological and social functions. George attends one or two meetings or events daily—up to fifteen each week—that counter feelings of stigmatization and isolation. Organizations replace losses from AIDS with whole new social networks. Support groups have also been one of the few treatments available to George (particularly before the development of protease inhibitors), one of the only steps he can take to help himself with the virus.

A support-group subculture has emerged which places a premium on discussing one's experiences. George and others feel they are supposed to talk about their illness, and that such talking can itself be therapeutic. Such groups become viewed as "solutions" in and of themselves, imbued with an almost magical sense of hope that is often a key ingredient in their overall appeal and effect.

Immersion in HIV-land occurs for numerous reasons. HIV-land accepts individuals along with their diagnosis. Wilma explained that in a group she can "come out" about her infection to others who will be accepting. In contrast, outside HIV-land she faces discrimination.

Basic knowledge about HIV also separates those in and outside this realm. Leonard Barber, a tall, thirty-one-year-old gay man with shaggy brown hair, lives in Westchester. "For the general, non-HIV infected community," he said, "the information is specialized, technical, and difficult to assimilate. At best, people have only a headline of knowledge. I end up having to explain why weird things show up and how the immune system breaks down. I react to what disabled people object to when others respond to them as somehow 'less than.' Some crucial element of my competence as a human being has been robbed by a medical condition.

To some I'm always first and foremost a person afflicted with my condition before I'm anything else.

"I don't like having to play catch-up with people who aren't informed. It's a lot simpler just not to raise it. People's lack of information is discouraging. If my HIV status comes out in the course of knowing somebody, their view of me almost always shifts. The issue, if not actually addressed, exists as a subtext. Occasionally I will choose not to approach somebody I might be interested in simply because I don't want to go through the rigmarole of talking about HIV. Sometimes I'm willing to walk people through their ignorance or anxiety, but other times not. Having to explain what I've had to say a million times before is not just boring. It makes me angry that I have to take time out to play science teacher, explaining the whole background of AIDS, chapters one through ten. I get pissed off: what in the hell right do you have to ignore this? I had to educate myself. Why should it be my responsibility to educate everybody else too? The concept of HIV disease as a continuum—that there's the sub-AIDS state of affairs called ARC—is not very well accepted, or understood." Others automatically see Leonard as having AIDS and dying, while he tries to see himself as 'living with' HIV.

"I'm also the first HIV-positive person that some in the non-HIV community have known, and they feel I'm not fighting hard enough. I don't like being their Big Brother, their first exposure to the illness, working their issues through for them and saying 'Everything's fine' and then going out and dying the next day."

The problems of the uninfected also begin to seem less important. As Maurice Bradford explained, "After giving up my career, it's very hard to relate to what some uninfected people perceive as difficulties in their lives. That interferes with my ability to be close to them. I'm not as empathetic as I used to be with what they're going through, most of which, from my perspective, seems rather trivial. One female friend of mine has been struggling for a year and a half over whether to move. The thought of just having a choice would really excite me.

"So I've had to weed out socially. For example, I needed some support—not a lot—from someone whom I thought was a close friend. But he fell through. I said, 'Fuck him.' After fifteen years he's no longer in my life. I'm not going to bring him along. Now is a time for paring, for reaping the seeds I've sown."

Not Singled Out

HIV-land provides a sense of being part of something larger and more ongoing than oneself. As Roy Gifford, the gay man about to retire, told me, "Initially I felt singled out to die young, having this monstrous, monumental disease. I didn't know anyone else with HIV. Since I've been diagnosed I've become reflective on my life—the good and the bad—and taken a philosophical view toward life and death. How can I accept the fact that I'm going to die, most likely at an early age? I try to view it in terms of history. Over the ages people have died: everybody has their trials. I'm not being singled out to die young. Millions of people have died in wars and other epidemics. When I see myself as a human being caught in a larger situation, I don't feel as alone. I'm part of this army, this group." Plagues aren't experienced only as individual medical events but as social and political. Individuals participate in and shape the larger phenomena, forming the constituent parts. Thus individual responses reflect and refract larger historical events.

Immersion in death occurs as part of this group's cohesiveness and identity. Many vividly described the visual and psychological impact of witnessing the deterioration and death of others. As Aaron Eliot described earlier, concerning his friend who died, "I began to understand how fragile we are, how important life is, and how we only have so much time on earth and should take best advantage of it."

Involvement in HIV-land becomes self-perpetuating as grief brings members closer. As George Sullivan said, "After my friend Tim passed away, I just had to spend a lot of time with people who knew him. There was no funeral in the city—his parents took his remains to Pennsylvania—so all I could do was talk with others who knew him too." For men and women who are alienated from the outside world, communication within HIV-land takes on added importance.

"Unfortunately, in the gay community people are often dead and you don't know it. They don't appear in the obit column of the *Times* unless somebody's around to make sure it gets in. I never knew their families and what happened when they died. I'll go to a party or bump into somebody and tell him about people he didn't know about, and he'll tell me about others. There's a grapevine."

Mutual losses help define and cement the community. Kerry Musgrove, who works for an AIDS organization, said, "I went to a Christmas party and in the middle of the dance floor was told that Jack died. I was very upset. He wasn't the great love of my life, but he was fun, and I liked him. Now I read the obituaries first thing every morning, so an asshole doesn't walk up to me at a party and tell me about someone I care about.

"Sometimes I cry even for people I never heard of. One guy was thirty and his parents put in the obituary, 'Tom died on a beautiful sunny day, swimming in his father's pool. He had AIDS and died of heart failure.' Obviously his parents loved him. Nobody wants to die, but it was a nice way to go, and nice to see his parents were taking care of him.

"I get angry at the Liberaces, those who won't reveal it even after they're dead. People could have learned from their deaths."

Deaths devastate injecting drug users as well as the gay community. As Jill Montgomery, who grew up in the inner city, said, "People in my neighborhood have been just disappearing, dropping dead like flies. 'Where's this girl?' 'Didn't you hear? She's in the hospital with PCP. . . . She died.' Whole neighborhoods are getting wiped out."

Living Rooms

Yet formal organizations in HIV-land are not for everyone. Although they serve multiple functions, not only educating but allowing patients to help others, and generally encourage those with a history of drug use to abstain, many patients dislike support groups and formal social structures. Aaron Eliot and others prefer informal relationships. "I've gotten involved a little with GMHC and AIDS organizations, but not support groups," he explained. "I forced myself to go to a group once, but I found it very depressing, and stopped. It wasn't for me. They bullshitted about this and that, and some people came in very sick and were getting sicker. I went for a short period, six weeks. But I started to feel better, and felt I didn't need it. It was too much grief.

"I also used to go to lunches at AIDS organizations. It wasn't a support group at a certain time with a certain number of people, but just being involved with people. The Living Room serves lunch a few times a week. I go and sit around, talk, and get the latest news.

"What has helped me most are friends. Without them I'd be a lost soul. We lean on each other and talk about our problems. They are wonderful, wonderful people! Most are gay, and all of them I've met since becoming sick. They are sick themselves, and a lot of them go back two or three years like myself. I speak to four or five people a day, every day.

"It has helped me talking to people who know what I'm going

through. I can speak with my sister and tell her this, that, and the other thing, but she still can't grasp it because it's not happening to her. One time she said to me, 'You're sixty-two, what do you expect?' That's very frustrating. Those who aren't infected don't know. They can't. They can sympathize but don't know the hell this disease brings. My friends going through it know.

"So I've formed my own support group of friends. I don't need a scheduled hour each week. I do it whenever I want. I pick up the phone and call this friend or that and just talk. It doesn't have to be only about AIDS. We talk about things in general—trips we've made. But a lot of it focuses on AIDS. What have you heard? Did you read this or that? Do you know about this procedure?

"All my friends now are sick. I have a two-page list here of names and phone numbers and addresses of friends. Every day I go down the sheets and call as many as I can, starting at the top or wherever I got to the day before. When I finish, I start all over again. I know of many, many people who have been affected."

Arlene Chambers, a forty-five-year-old African-American woman with a past history of injecting drug use, said, "Everything in a support group is supposed to be confidential. But it gets out. I've seen it happen. Someone got up in AA and revealed he was HIV positive. Three minutes later the whole neighborhood knew. I've never liked support groups. I don't like to talk about my problems to people I don't know."

Many dislike support groups for other reasons. Jenny Singer: "My support group at first made me feel a lot better—I wasn't alone. They understood and could joke and make fun of it. We could have a good laugh. But I didn't want to get close to more people who were going to die because many of my friends had already passed away." Individual therapy rather than groups may sometimes be indicated. "One evening I opened up the group and was using it, expressing how upset I was that a friend was dying. The group fell silent. The leader finally said, 'I think you should really bring that up with your individual therapist.' That was it. They went on talking and making jokes about something else. I felt I had brought a bomb into the room."

HIV-land also provides various rituals of mourning. Memorial services organized by friends honor many gay men with AIDS who were unmarried and estranged from their families of origin. Before they die, some patients throw parties for themselves. Guests, familiar with such events, line up to "say goodbye" to the dying man before leaving the party. Members of HIV-land who sew and display massive paneled AIDS quilts also creatively memorialize the lives of the deceased, periodically blanketing the Washington Mall and other public areas. Hundreds of thousands of people then walk among and view the panels, each different and unique like the departed individuals there remembered. The quilts themselves embody tradition, patchwork quilts being part of preindustrial Americana. Here, though, they convey parts of the individual symbolically into the future, using photos—on film and silk screen—bits of jeans, denim jackets, favorite hats, and other possessions embroidered in and thus incorporated into the future, to be viewed well after the individual's death.

Acting Up

In HIV-land disagreements persist over politics and political action. Matt Winchell, a thirty-three-year-old gay man, now works full-time for ACT-UP, the AIDS Coalition to Unleash Power, an organization founded by Larry Kramer and others that advocates for the interests of HIV-infected individuals through political action, including demonstrations or "zaps" against government agencies, pharmaceutical companies, and other organizations Matt, tall with short cropped blond hair, wore brown boots, jeans, and an unbuttoned flannel shirt with a white T-shirt underneath. For years, before finding out he was HIV positive, he had struggled without success in film and video. "Initially I was very angry about having to worry about this illness and being unable to direct my anger at anything. All I could do was wander around on the street, pissed off in general. Now I feel the government contributes to a lot of the problems I have to face, for example about AZT. The government's handling of this epidemic has been nothing short of criminal. Luckily I can target my anger now, so it's less frustrating." On his job he researches and writes reports on standard and alternative treatments for HIV. "I love my job," he says, "and often work after hours. I have finally found my calling."

ACT-UP has become an integral part of Matt's identity and his social and political life, and serves multiple functions for him. "An ACT-UP meeting is a great place to get a date—a roomful of good-looking men, for whom being HIV positive isn't an impediment. I assume that most of the people there are HIV positive themselves." Yet he also derides the social dynamics of the organization. "There are cliques like in high school: the crew team, the nerds, and the politicos." He feels excluded from some of these groups but has found a niche for himself in others. Factions riddle this segment of HIV-land, drawn together by crisis.

For Matt the possibility of death has triggered this radical political response. In the 1960s the Vietnam draft and the threat of dying in Southeast Asia galvanized young people in America to fight "the system" and become activists in "the movement." AIDS rekindled that activism. Death and politics again come together as Matt and others respond to private grievances in a larger public forum. The possibility of imminent death diminishes their risk in combating the government, speaking out, even getting arrested. Matt and others now define themselves as representative of the epidemic. Matt described "lying down on the street in front of the NIH, blocking entry to the driveway. The police had to carry us away and we got parking tickets, but it felt good putting my body literally on the line." Politicization also changes the self, providing a new identity as "activist"—a sense that one has the ability, the legitimacy, the strength to speak and be heard.

Yet others dislike ACT-UP's dynamics. Roy Gifford went to a few meetings but complained, "They're anarchic, and very long and torturous, starting at seven and going to past eleven-thirty. Being in a meeting with eight hundred positive people is very empowering. But fighting the bureaucracy and talking about death all the time deplete me. The physical deterioration of many of the people also depresses me. Moreover, no matter how much we do, thousands of hurdles remain. So my first priority now is my own health." ACT-UP's "anarchy" results from several factors, including a rapid turnover of leaders because of illness and death. The group also adheres to an open, egalitarian style, impeding organizational structure and hierarchy.

George Sullivan instead seeks other avenues within HIV-land. To take to the streets and risk arrest lie far from his previous activities at Harvard and on Wall Street. He also views politics with cynicism and resignation. Matt and others who get involved tend to have felt more enfranchised in the political process to start with.

ACT-UP is a distinctly American response. It was begun in this country, but chapters have sprung up abroad, with mixed results. ACT-UP groups in Ireland, Japan, and Thailand, for instance, face very different cultural and political obstacles. None has been as successful as the American entity.

ACT-UP intersects with other HIV-land organizations in various ways. Matt told me he was "the only one who attends ACT-UP meetings on Monday nights and the Healing Circle [a holistic health group] on Wednesday nights. ACT-UP looks down on the Healing Circle, which is apolitical and emphasizes making yourself healthy rather than fighting other people about the system. But I don't like the Healing Circle's constant 'me, me, me' position either." Each group addresses different aspects of his life. Personal backgrounds and needs shape organizational involvements.

Those affected with HIV segregate into groups through self-selection. Gay men such as Matt form the majority of ACT-UP's ranks. IDUs such as Alfie Montoya tend to be more involved in other organizations, such as Momentum, which supplies free meals. Yet overlaps occur. Many women have joined ACT-UP. George, with a past alcohol problem, now attends a twelve-step program.

Still, tensions persist. Roy doesn't like GMHC anymore because "it's become a junkie haven, and everyone I used to know there is dead now." Moreover, HIV-land can never fully replace the many losses that occur. Jenny lamented, "A lot of people are missing from my life now and can't be replaced. I can make a bunch of new friends, but it doesn't replace the feeling of people that were in my life. I'm entirely surrounded by death."

The House of Death

Residences for HIV-infected individuals raise these issues acutely, yielding both benefits and problems. Jill Montgomery explained, "I live in a house of positive people. I'm surrounded by people who are all HIV. It's good and it's bad. Good because we don't have to work that issue through. We accept each other for what we are, support each other, and can talk about our fears. But it's sad when one of them gets sick. People cry.

"People also cough and have symptoms all around me while I'm trying to fight. So I'm beginning to wonder about these surroundings. I did well all these years not around other HIV people. I'm wondering if it helps to be around them—emotionally too. A young girl, twenty-something, had been there and died. I've seen pictures of her. One of the girls she was close to asked me to go with her to the funeral. I didn't know the girl that died. I thought, 'How could it affect me?' So I went. I sat down and looked at the coffin. I could see that the girl who had died was young. She didn't look real. I got a headache and wondered, why am I feeling this? When my husband got killed, I couldn't see his coffin or his body. Now, I felt, 'God, is this going to happen to me?' The girl's father cried and they were saying she had been looking good and it had just happened. All of a sudden her kidney and her liver had kicked in. In less than a week she went from being healthy. Reality slapped me. I thought, 'My God. She was like me.' I saw how vicious this disease could be. One minute I can see a healthy person like me and, God forbid, next week she'll be dead. It was a shock. I made up my mind that I'm not going to go to nobody's funeral I don't know. I don't go to many, but it has to be somebody I know. Even then, I don't know how I'd feel."

Dede Alwin, a single thirty-six-year-old African-American woman and former injecting drug user, said, "My residence is like a hospital. They bring in really sick people. Some are bedridden. It didn't feel like a hospital when I first got there. But now I'm around too many sick people. Everybody always talks about sickness. I don't like hearing about it." Reminders of death are difficult to avoid.

"There's also no privacy," Dede went on, "and I can't really get the rest I want. It's a hole—twenty-eight people, all HIV positive, who can't seem to mind their own business. They're always trying to learn somebody else's business instead of bettering themselves. They're skinny, look bad, talk about everybody else, and don't care for themselves. Misery loves company. They're like kids tattle-telling: this person is getting high or doing this or that. I stay in my room and don't even bother going downstairs. I'm not the type to sit and cry, oh I'm dying . . . I'm dying. I don't even think about it. The only time it pops in my head that I have AIDS is when I have to go to the doctor. The other twenty-eight days of the month I don't think about it. And being in this residence is a constant reminder. Certain people just sit there day in and day out, don't go anywhere or do anything, and always complain and whine. Nothing is good enough for them. It's like an old-age home. I want to move.

"The staff also drive new cars. They don't want to deal with a bunch of dope fiends. They figure we didn't know any better and will be grateful for a roof over our heads." Her resentment in part reflects her disfranchisement and discomfort in having to depend on such an institution.

For Roger Babson, a forty-two-year-old gay man now living in an AIDS residence, ethnic and class differences exacerbate these problems. "A lot of people at my residence are not my cup of tea. I don't feel friendly toward them. They talk street talk. So I pretty much keep to myself. I'm more comfortable in my room anyway. I don't have to deal with the outside world. When I moved there, I thought: this is the end. This is where I will waste away. I'll just stay in this bed and cover myself with the blankets. It will go from here to worse. It was a major effort to take a shower and get dressed. A lot of people, including myself, view it as a House of Death. It's putting the cows out to pasture, saying goodbye. Just before I moved in, a receptionist at one HIV organization asked me my address. I told him where I was moving. He said, 'Oh, you poor thing!'

"It took some adjustment for me. The first couple of days there I didn't eat and bought my food elsewhere. I didn't like having to share the dining room with people I didn't know or like. They looked sick or had teeth missing. Three-quarters were black. Very few were white. When I finally started eating there, I kept to myself, sitting alone at a dining table. But after a while I started listening to other conversations and found there were some nice people, with intelligence and good senses of humor. It's gotten much better because I started judging people by their individual qualities rather than as a group. It took four or five months. Some people I've come to like. We talk about each other's health. I see it more as a family now. I feel warm and loving toward them. They may be the last people I know." In these ways, residences can become all-encompassing—almost "total institutions," in Erving Goffman's use of the phrase.

HIV-land improves many lives, in part because they have been so deplorable and unfulfilled. Infection commonly occurs against a backdrop of previous rejection and isolation; and poverty and drug and alcohol abuse frequently affect more than one member of a family. Gloria Higgens, for example, a forty-eight-year-old African-American woman now living in an AIDS residence, has her own room for the first time in years. When I met with her, she sat on the edge of her bed wearing a freshly washed pair of jeans and a bright red kerchief. "Before, I was living in abandoned buildings and on the street," she told me. "I used to sleep in the park in front of the United Nations. People who worked there would sometimes walk over and give me old sweaters and clothes. Now for the first time I have a telephone and a TV."

Matt, too, has established more satisfying relationships than before he was infected. Through ACT-UP he entered his first committed long-term relationship. "If I didn't now, I don't know when I would. I used to date a lot of good-looking guys who were fun but never stayed in my life more than a few weeks or months. I may only have a few years to live. I realized I'd better find someone soon—get serious, grow up.

"I used to think being gay was bad. I felt different and weird and didn't understand why. Since I started working with other gay people, I've felt the best I ever have about myself—no longer an ugly failure." Matt and others illustrate how one's sense of self can be shaped by social organizations and environment.

Many injecting drug users undergo particularly marked changes. Eddie Lourdes, a Latino man now off drugs, said, "I feel like a new man. I hang out with people who would never have even talked to me before. People with careers—cops, firemen, and businessmen." HIV thus fosters equality across social classes. The HIV community helps these men and women change their views of themselves not only as HIV positive but in other fundamental ways.

HIV-land helps provide for redemption, such that being infected isn't necessarily a form of hell. Gloria Higgens said, "AIDS made me realize that life is worth living. Sometimes now when I wake up in the morning I feel like a normal person. HIV has been a blessing in disguise—a second chance."

Yet individuals enter this world of disease and become "professional patients" to differing degrees. Leonard Barber, living in Westchester where he runs a gardening business, said, "I decided early on that unless a serious illness intrudes and makes everything else superfluous, I'm not going to make my life about HIV. If in order to save my life I had to abandon everything else, it wouldn't be worth it. People shut down their lives to keep themselves well. But a lot of that is just magic. There might be a universe in which magic is possible, but I don't think this is one."

Leonard is less involved in the HIV community, in part because he has had fewer losses. "I've been relatively lucky compared to a lot of people. I'm not one of those who have had ninety-eight people in their address book die. Less than ten people I've known relatively well have died, though in the last couple of years the death rate has gone up in my circle of friends and acquaintances." He also has remained living where he had been for several years before being tested—outside the city. HIV-land has geographic as well as social boundaries.

Infected men and women create their own alternative universe which replaces the one they had. This new realm arises from loss and discrimination and provides new connections to others with the illness both now and in the future—a sense that one is not alone. Barriers of information, geography, and interest separate this land from the outside, and infected men and women enter to varying degrees—full-time or part-time, formally or informally, politically or socially. Tensions arise too, and HIV-land is not for everyone or joined without ambivalence. But this community nonetheless offers great benefits that can outweigh its costs.

FOUR

HIV-Land: *The Language*

HIV-LAND ALSO PROVIDES a new language which helps to organize and make sense of the illness and resulting confusion. The HIV community shapes its own conceptions of the virus, the epidemic, treatment, prognosis, and the health care system. As George Sullivan said, "At a lot of specialized HIV-positive AA meetings, we don't talk about booze, we talk about medicine like a bunch of frocked or unfrocked doctors. We tell each other, 'Do this, do that'—practical and paramedical things about getting rashes taken care of, and about doctors, nurses, benefits, and the virus."

Finding Words

HIV-land offers familiar terms and metaphors that can be applied to this unusual disease. HIV is difficult partly because it can be invisible, intangible, and mysterious. As Eddie Lourdes said, it's like "a bad omen—as if someone put a bad wish on me, bad vibes." The disease is also protean and not organ specific—"a lit-

tle bit of everything, depending on how your immune system han-
dles it."

HIV-land reframes prognoses as well as the diagnosis itself.
George Sullivan explained, "Today I say that HIV is like diabetes.
I keep saying that so I'll hear it myself, along with the friends I'm
reassuring. We in HIV-land try to reassure each other: 'it's a manageable disease and the cure's around the corner, and there are
these vaccines.'" Comparisons often arise with diabetes, an illness
that can be survived for decades if properly managed.

Others struggle to find an appropriate category. "What does
'chronic' mean?" Dede Alwin, who complained about her residence, asked. "Is that an illness that can't be cured?"

Problems arise in establishing an appropriate time frame for and
adjusting to death, and to the loss of the future. George explained,
"In HIV-land we learn to live now, not in the future or the past,
and try to take advantage of every single day. This is excellent HIV
advice, central to living in HIV-land. HIV has made me come to
grips with mortality and with things that I've been putting off because 'I've got a lifetime.' One hundred years ago, with TB and
other diseases, everybody felt that way. But now it's just us here in
HIV-land."

Within HIV-land a variety of metaphors have gained currency.
Chiefly the virus evokes a range of war allusions, spurred in part
by the language of immune functioning itself. Physicians refer to
the body's "defenses." "Killer" and "helper T-cells" are the official
medical terms for the types of blood cells involved in HIV. In HIV-
land this language becomes elaborated. Maurice Bradford, the
health care administrator, told me, "My cells are mobilizing
against the virus as it attacks me. I want to do everything I can to
aid the troops of cells inside my body." Matt described himself as
"besieged by more and more little things here and there—diarrhea, sores in my mouth. But I am proud of the way my body has
fought back."

The epidemic becomes compared to war because of other, broader effects as well, particularly the widespread dying that results. George said, "Not since World War II—which I remember as a kid, putting pins in a map of the world hanging in the kitchen— or Vietnam, have so many young people died all at once." In fact, San Francisco has lost four times more young men to AIDS than to World Wars I and II, Korea, and Vietnam combined. In war, however, families and governments praise soldiers for fighting, and decorate warriors as heroes. For most soldiers, the threat of death ends at some point, and civilian life resumes. They or their survivors also receive pensions and other benefits for years to come. AIDS provides none of these compensations.

Inner-city residents draw analogies more specific to street warfare. Some imagine an inner city existing within their body. To make this aggressive but sometimes invisible disease more tangible, the virus becomes reified and frequently anthropomorphized. Alfie Montoya, the former injecting drug user who first became concerned about HIV when he started medications, had spent years on the street trying to elude police because of drug-related activities. He had also served time in prison. "AIDS attacks you from the inside out," he explained, "and by your immune system getting beaten up, allowing various illnesses within you to flare up. The virus is small and weak, but slick, and disguises itself to try to fool you. It watches for slipups and spots any negative thoughts, even if they're in the back of your mind. It's like combat. If I show my enemy I am not scared, he'll doubt and weaken himself. That's when you overcome the enemy. If you don't think about this virus being such a strong thing, and aren't scared of it, you're going to gain strength within you. If I start doing things I'm not supposed to, I'll wake it up. It's telling me, 'I'm going to lay down and rest as long as you eat the proper food and don't do drugs. Don't disturb me, or I'll act like a monster, and take you out.' If I give the virus the slightest idea that I'm not sure about myself and think this virus is stronger than me, this virus is going to get over on me." Street warfare clearly relies on psychological intimidation.

"At one time I thought fighting for my life meant defending myself on the street. Now I know that you don't have to go to war to fight for your life. People fight for their lives in different ways. But I don't give this virus the opportunity to take me over. This virus is a small weak thing. Nobody would expect such a little thing to be so strong and devastating. But it's very, very cunning, able to change from one second to another. One minute it's this, the next minute that. That's one of the reasons finding a cure is so hard"— which scientifically is correct. But Alfie goes on, viewing the virus in terms he understands. "The virus disguises itself as a duplicate of a person's cells, using the same code to enter the bloodstream. Once in there, it gets into the mainstream of the computer and has access to what it wants. It programs the computer: instead of sending out T-4 cells, it sends out more viruses. It's like a spy, an agent. It passes for the same kind of agent that is supposed to watch the designated area. Once in there, nothing can identify it. Once it comes out, it changes back into its original disguise and attacks more T-cells. It camouflages the cell and makes the cell know nothing.

"The virus also knows where to go to break down your immune system and take all your defenses away. It knows your system. It goes for the T-cells that fight off infections—your main source of artillery. It has such a good disguise that it gets into the T-cells and is difficult to pin down. It knows what to attack and leaves alone other things that are not so devastating to it and won't do nothing to the virus. It knows that if I attack T-cells, all the rest are helpless. Once I get them, I have control of everything." Alfie too has been sly on the street, and at one point he failed to tell his drug counselor that he had tested positive.

Alfie also views his disease as similar to addiction and withdrawal, or "going cold turkey. AZT is not strong enough to wipe the virus out completely, and the virus has a way of coming back to life. Once you take a certain dose on a consistent basis, the AZT maintains the virus. But once you stop, the virus might wake up and come back ten times stronger than before. Nature is like that. Nature knows. The clouds know. When they ain't got water inside, they're nice and white, and when they start absorbing water they turn gray. When they got a lot of water inside they crash and collapse." Anthropomorphic understandings—teleo-logic, and imbuing the virus with intention and will—help provide explanations.

Gregory Colson, a former injecting drug user who served in Vietnam, sees the virus as if it were ammunition, bullets, "a bunch of different viruses hitting you at one shot in your immune sys-tem."

For Aaron Eliot, HIV resembles war on a grander level, all en-compassing. "There are many aspects: on the job, with life issues, questions of 'Why am I gay?' and 'Why me?' It's like the Persian Gulf War, which happened right after I tested positive. This is my war."

In a modern high-technology society, images of machines arise to make sense of biological processes. "The body has an engine that has to be as fine-tuned and perfectly running as possible," Matt Winchell explained. "That means no gunk can go in there— no junk food, alcohol, or cigarettes. To keep that engine running at peak capacity I allow only exercise, good food, and taking care of myself."

Roy Gifford said, "My body is a P24 antibody-producing ma-chine—a factory." He sees the process as mechanistic, separate from himself and his will.

In these responses we can see how the virus becomes imbued with cognition. Technically a virus is not even alive—it is not a cell, it cannot reproduce by itself outside of a host cell, and has no metabolism and certainly no nervous system. Yet as Gerry Galvez, whom the orderly had initially visited in the hospital, said, "It's a bug inside me that just won't go away. It stays in my system and doesn't start reacting or activating until it decides to. I don't know when it's going to attack. I'm angry that the virus doesn't give you a warning, or say, 'Guess what. I'm gonna attack you next week.' I've been in meetings with twenty people and a couple of months later four or five were missing."

She also sees the virus as having bodily functions. "It's parasitic like cancer, and eats up everything that can help my system." Thus she too minimizes the randomness involved by ascribing willfulness to the virus itself. The virus has a system and a plan even if she doesn't know what they are.

Injecting drug users see the virus as a drug too—a foreign material inside the body, entering through the same route as drugs and having as wide-ranging effects. Arlene Chambers, an IDU, told me, "I don't think drugs affect HIV, unless you reinfect yourself using a dirty needle, adding more virus to your body"—a dose effect, similar to that of drugs.

Prison metaphors also help in understanding AIDS. Gregory Colson, after serving in Vietnam, spent time in jail because of drug use. "I now have a death sentence," he said, describing HIV, "but don't know the date." Prison, like chronic disease, restricted him for a prolonged period of time. In both situations, external powers have controlled him against his will.

"Plague" metaphors arise, providing precedents for destruction wreaked by an infectious disease. The term "Black Death" conjures up hellish and macabre images which may also be applied to AIDS. Jenny Singer and others associate HIV with "leprosy" and feel like "lepers," ostracized for fear of contagion. (The term *leper* arose as a medical diagnosis and then for centuries was employed as a metaphor in other nonmedical situations. Now, with HIV, the word has both metaphoric and literal connotations.)

Those from rural rather than urban environments rely more on metaphors drawn from nature. Roy Gifford, about to retire, grew up in New Jersey, near the Palisades, and was trained in biology. "If I drew a picture of HIV," he told me, "it would be the 'Green Blob' in a very low-budget, low-quality horror movie, squidging along, sliding down a hill like a lava flow. It keeps moving like the glacier that came down and carved the Hudson Valley and the Palisades." He sees glaciers as unstoppable, uncontrollable natural forces and believes the virus will eventually kill him and others—a whole geological and social region.

Those angry about having been infected sexually see the virus more in sexual terms. Maurice Bradford, the health care administrator, refers to the virus as "the little fucker." As a gay man, he was infected by getting "fucked," and the virus, an unwanted partner in his sexual life, has "fucked things up" for him.

He and others also internalize the virus. "It is in me," he continues, "as if my body is self-destructing." The process is inside and part of him, an extension of who he is. His body is attacking itself as a result of his actions—tinged for him with guilt. His moral view of himself molds his view of the physiologic process inside him.

The virus and the illness thus becomes parts of one's identity. Wilma and others refer to themselves as "being HIV" and say about one another that he or she "is HIV," as if the person *is* the virus.

Reading Signs

HIV-land interprets not only the virus itself but signs, symptoms, and markers of the illness's progression, revealing the anxiety that surrounds the threat of death. For example, members of HIV-land discuss at length T-cells, sharing one another's results, to learn how to make sense of these laboratory findings. Before the epidemic, physicians knew little about the clinical meanings of these cells. Now, as Maurice Bradford said, "My T-cell count was low and then got better—a common pattern. Then it got worse—another common pattern." He has acquired in his mind firm, expected ranges of values. Wilma "announced in my group that my T-cells went up, and everyone applauded."

Yet though T-cells mark the progression of HIV infection, confusion remains. With little or no clinical change, these counts rise or fall, death now hovering nearby or temporarily fleeing. T-cells, representing either a protection against or a worsening of the disease, become the focus of fear and conflict, enshrouded by a complex web of meanings and imbued with special, almost magical significance. Laboratory tests became anthropomorphized. As Maurice joked, though melancholically, "I have eight T-cells—so few I can invite them all over for dinner, or name them and remember the names."

Unfortunately T-cells act independently of one's will. As with recipients of transplant organs, who similarly concretize their illness to make an otherwise ambiguous and mystifying state more objective, those infected with HIV seek tangible ways of understanding these cells. T-cells are, after all, both part of oneself yet independent.

Wilma and others also see T-cells as mediating agents between themselves and the disease. "When I started taking better care of myself," she observed, "my T-count went up." Alfie Montoya commented, "I'm fine now except for my T-cells," distinguishing himself from them and maintaining a view of himself as essentially okay despite their condition.

Why do others have fewer or more cells? Gloria Higgens, in the AIDS residence with her own room for the first time in years, has a high T-count and concluded, "I must have a less powerful strain." A lot of people who have died got infected after I did, and

I'm wondering if the virus I got wasn't as strong." George Sullivan said, "I must have 'whore's blood.' My body must have built up immunity through repeated small exposures."

Yet bafflement continues. "With only eight T-cells, I should be dead," Maurice said. "Yet here I am. So who knows? I know someone who has *no* T-cells. How can you walk around and have none?" He maintains an ironic distance yet eagerly seeks and monitors these numbers in order to quantify this often ill-defined disease. Infected individuals, detesting the virus and wanting more T-cells, also joke about the former more than the latter.

Of note, scientists have switched to using the term "CD4 counts" instead of "T-cells." Yet common parlance in HIV-land has not shifted. After all, T-cells are more tangible than CD4 counts, referring to entities rather than to abstract "counts."

Pole Reversals

To help its inhabitants make sense of their experience, HIV-land gives meanings not only to relevant medical terms but to other words. The words *positive* and *negative* themselves become redefined. As Alfie Montoya said, "I don't consider myself sick. I believe a person creates his own shit—meaning illness. If you think sick, you're going to get sick. If you think healthy, you remain healthy. You create your own negative and positive."

In fact, he and others reverse the meanings of these two terms. Jill Montgomery now says, "I try to surround myself only with positive people. At my residence there are negative people who bring me down. I try to avoid them." Wilma Smith tries "to maintain a positive view of life, a positive lifestyle, and a positive frame of mind." Thus "being positive" is not being "sick," "contaminated," or "ugly" but "optimistic" and "hopeful." Conversely, "being negative" now embodies undesirable characteristics of being depressed, angry, or hostile. This switch in polarities destigmatizes positivity and mitigates the sense of being "taboo."

For some, positivity takes on a spiritual dimension. Olana Ramirez, who feared disintegration, explained, "My spiritual is my positive side. My negative side is the nonspiritual. It's the side that doesn't care, that doesn't want to feel, that wants to sedate. It hurts and wants to hurt. I don't like that side. I have my 'good thinking' and my 'stinking thinking.'" In her book *Purity and Danger* the anthropologist Mary Douglas describes an essential tension in cultures between purity and pollution. For the inhabitant of HIV-land, negotiating a position between these poles becomes a central task, and individuals redefine themselves in this new social and medical context.

Yet "thinking positively" nonetheless connotes different things to different people. Alfie, who sees the virus as "slick," wants to take a trip but doesn't have the money. "If it doesn't come, it was not meant for me to go. If it happens, it happens: that's what I mean by 'positive mental attitude,'"—avoiding unrealistic hopes and expectations, and accepting events as they occur. "I really don't want to stop smoking cigarettes, even though I know they're not really healthy. So I'm not *super*positive." Positivity thus also has gradations, and individuals choose how positive to be—some are more positive than others.

Because the behaviors that transmit the virus have been labeled by society as taboo, redefinition of the self becomes crucial. The censure of homosexuality, drug use, and unchaste sexual relationships lead many who learn they are HIV positive to feel guilty. Consequently HIV-land seeks to change perceptions of the disease among its members and others. HIV-land explicitly challenges the notion that the infected are "victims" or even "patients." Rather, they are merely PWAs—people "with" or "living with" HIV or AIDS. PWAs feel the term *victim* adds emotional and moral weight and suggests helplessness, passivity, and failure to be in charge of one's life. They value "empowerment," not "victimization."

Yet not all wish to avoid the term *victim*. Many are quite happy to gain whatever added attention, recognition, and benefits it may offer. As Wilma says, "If I had received the virus through a transfusion, it wouldn't have been my fault. I would have been a victim. I could have just focused on 'you did this to me.' Being a victim is more acceptable than my behavior and my lifestyle in my past." Feeling like a victim allows many to focus their anger and avoid blaming themselves for possibly having infected others.

Pills and Potions

To reduce fears and uncertainty, and offer a sense of control over the possibility of death, HIV-land frames discussions about medications, vaccines, and cures. Patients compare their medication regimens and resulting clinical courses, making decisions about treatment and becoming in effect their own physicians. Dede Alwin, who complained about her AIDS residence, never completed high school but now compares and evaluates details of pharmacology. "I've talked with people on Datzol only twice a day who are doing fine. So I realized that I don't need to take it four times a day as my doctor said. Since then I've been doing better." Although new treatments are continually being approved, the issues expressed here concerning medications reveal important underlying attitudes that remain highly relevant, especially as newer drugs demand even more complicated regimens.

Members of HIV-land question and restructure the doctor-patient relationship. In the absence of certainty, decisions about AZT, for example, become matters of faith. As George Sullivan said, "I'm not a believer in AZT. I like the concept but not the consequences. The side effects are too severe—anemia, pancreatitis, lymphoma, and bone marrow malfunction." The high stakes and relatively low level of existing knowledge create believers and non-believers, as if AZT were a matter of magic or religion—which it indeed often becomes.

Analogies and metaphors try to make sense of medications. As Carrie Serano, a former IDU, said, "AZT puts the virus to sleep," though whether the virus here ends up dead—like a dog—or merely dormant remains ambiguous.

Non-Western approaches and viewpoints become popular. HIV-land, having set itself up as an alternative to the medical establish-ment, endorses alternative treatments and approaches. To deal with his body's reactions to the virus regardless of his will, Matt Win-chell adopts a holistic sense of his body and an antimedical stance. He sits in his office surrounded by thin, dull, reused plastic bags stuffed with dried brown leaves and branches of medicinal plants which he boils daily for tea. "Clearly my body has been keeping this thing in check now for a long time. I'm very proud of my body for doing that. I haven't taken AZT because 'if something's not broken, don't fix it.' If I dropped below two hundred T-cells consis-tently, I would have done AZT a while ago. My gut instinct about AZT from people I've known who've taken it is negative. Even tak-ing Bactrim would be a very strong message to myself that I no longer trust my body: you're obviously going to lose, so take this medicine. I have to tell my body, 'Come on, body, slug it out. You can beat 'em.' I want to be able to fight this thing on my own.

"I've always been a fighter, and letting doctors put toxic drugs in my body is stressful. My body is me—my essence, what I am. I have great confidence in my body, which means I have confidence in myself, even though I still abuse myself by finding fault with and criticizing, worrying, and hating myself.

"I feel victorious as a survivor when I go into a bar and every-body there wants me. I was the nerd of my high school; everybody thought I was an idiot, and nobody would touch me with a ten-foot pole. I worked out, got in shape, cut my hair right, and learned how to look attractive. Now they're all dying for me. One of my biggest dreams since I was twelve years old has been to have twenty more pounds of muscle, and I did it last year." For him and others, the gym becomes a central locale in HIV-land. Exercise wards off illness and creates an appearance of health and strength.

"The fact that my body isn't functioning depresses me a lot more than being HIV positive," Matt adds. His diseased body deeply disturbs him. Same-sex attractions having triggered his identification of himself as gay, he now seeks affirmation as a gay man through his body.

Limitations in medical treatments fuel his holistic beliefs. "I asked the doctor if there was anything that could be done for the virus. He said, 'Virtually no.' I said, 'That's all I wanted to know. Running around town to find a medical treatment won't do anything. Thank you for allowing me some peace.'" Matt likes the certainty of knowing—even if it is that no treatment exists. He and others also view doctors and researchers skeptically as "them," the other. "I don't believe they will find a cure that would alleviate all that has already happened to me."

HIV-land disseminates information about alternative options, weeding out and comparing various treatment options, but the possibilities can overwhelm. "A friend asked me if I'd heard about bitter lemons," Aaron Eliot told me. "He's squeezing them up and putting them in a blender—the latest thing. There are so many 'latest things.' It's crazy out there. There is so much information and confusion. I don't see how anybody can understand what's going on."

Once one is infected, the reasons to take medication, at least before the recent advent of protease inhibitors, have been less compelling than in other disorders. Jill reported, "They tell me I need Pentamidine, but I don't believe it. It just doesn't sit right in my mind. I can't see continuously taking something as potent as this drug to stop or prevent something that other people who have been taking this medicine got anyway. You can't prove to me that it will stop or prevent me from getting something. It doesn't work. It's not normal to take medication three times a day for the rest of my life for something it doesn't cure. And I don't want to depend on nothing. I depended on heroin and cocaine for twenty-three years, and I just can't see going back there.

"I've seen AZT bring people a new kind of hope. And then, eventually, they all come off it. I saw a guy who looked like he was dead—emaciated, hair lost. He took AZT for a while and it gave him hope. But I believe that what helped him was not the AZT but the fact that they *told* him it would help, because when he came off it last year he kept doing well and never reverted to that person he was."

Others, pro-AZT, criticize the skeptics. Olana Ramirez observed, "I know people who sell their medication. Three months ago a girl told me, 'I know where you can get $25 for the big bottles.' Here you're getting something for free through Medicaid to save your life. It's crazy to turn around and sell it in the street, and just throw your life away like that. Especially for $25, which won't even take care of a flower when you die."

Medications, given their complex and ambiguous effects, also become anthropomorphized. As Gerry Galvez said, "AZT helps your immune system and T-cell count in the beginning. But then after three or four months, it no longer boosts your system and just hangs out." Thus medication too is viewed not only in human but in *familiar* human terms—it "hangs out," as do Gerry and her acquaintances.

Opinions vary as to the possibility of a definitive cure. Jenny Singer said, "I feel they will come up with a cure. At one time they thought there was never going to be a cure for syphilis or TB. People died from TB and got locked up or sent away. So I feel that when I do die, it won't be from AIDS but something else. I have had chronic asthma since I was small. I even got left back in school because of it. So I always had a fear of that."

The possibility of a cure thus carries a wide range of meanings and associations. But some doubt that if a cure were developed, it would be made available to them. Vaccines too take on various meanings. Mitchell Walters, a thirty-six-year-old Caucasian injecting drug user, said, "I'll be glad when they come out with a shot they could give to a woman I fall in love with so I could have sex and kids with her and not have to worry about the disease."

Puns

Humor plays a critical role in this community and facilitates conversations about different aspects of the epidemic. The term *HIV-land* itself embodies a degree of wit. Jokes flourish here partly because an audience exists to appreciate them. Freud, in *Jokes and Their Relationship to the Unconscious*, argues that humor reveals key characteristics of unconscious thought processes. Within HIV-land, sarcasm prevails that allows for expression of bitterness and rage. Irony also emerges from a long tradition of gay camp, mocking institutions felt to be homophobic or unsympathetic. Inverted meanings have long existed in gay culture. Farce also thrives in HIV-land. Several years ago a play opened in Los Angeles entitled *AIDS: The Musical*.

Black humor can ease anxieties resulting from the threat of the virus. As part of an experimental protocol, Roy Gifford, the gay man forced to retire, must inject himself with a syringe four times a day. "I refer to this as my works," he says. "Shooting up. My beeper went off in a restaurant, and I sat there trying to figure out what to do—how to prepare a syringe discreetly in a dirty men's room. I decided to prepare it on the table on the white tablecloth, in the middle of a conversation. I just pulled out my stuff and said, 'Excuse me, I have to play with my works.' At the other tables, people's jaws dropped. I just thought to myself, 'If you only knew. This is New York. Get used to it, girls.' "

Roy's humor gives voice to his otherwise unexpressed pain, sadness, fear, and rage over being contaminated and thus having to confront stigma and death. "I also got from a lab some 'Biohazard' stickers and put one on my knapsack. I should be responsible when carrying around a hypodermic needle. If somebody steals my backpack and gets a hold of my syringe, they should be warned that it's contaminated. They've been forewarned. "

HIV-land embraces a range of terms and conceptual frameworks for understanding the virus and its consequences. Individuals search desperately to comprehend diagnoses, prognoses, viral mechanisms, immunological defenses, disease markers and processes, medications, epidemiological trends, and changes in identity. Patients "read" these phenomena, making interpretations, fitting raw experiences into categories, and drawing on metaphors from the environment and from personal and societal history. Analogies are drawn from military combat, street warfare, prison, factories, machines, computers, addictions, and better-understood diseases and biological processes. Confronted by a new experience, these established images help make HIV familiar and hence more manageable. This vocabulary helps patients grasp the experience of being infected, given the uncertainties and fears that result from loss and rejection. The enemy must be concretized in order to know how to deal with it.

The groups, organizations, and interactions of HIV-land propagate and share these terms, which in turn draw individuals further into the HIV community. This language helps individuals not only make sense of the infection but recreate themselves and their worlds.

FIVE

Higher Powers

BESIDES SEEKING a new social order through HIV-land, patients search for spiritual connection and a renewed sense of moral order. Spirituality, drawn from different sources, serves a variety of functions and incorporates a wide range of beliefs. Yet such beliefs can also pose difficulties, as doubts, obstacles, and often decades of atheism or agnosticism must first be overcome.

To the Saint of Hopeless Causes

Jason Gillian, a thirty-five-year-old gay man, was raised Roman Catholic. Although he relies on this religious tradition, he also revises it to meet his new needs. He grew up in a small town in rural Indiana, "the hinterlands. As soon as I knew there was a New York, I knew that was where I wanted to be," he said. "I finally moved here when I was twenty-one." Now he works in an antique store. He met me after work, wearing a navy suit, black loafers, a white shirt, and a silver and red tie. He had neatly trimmed light brown hair and bright blue eyes. He fit easily among the businessmen on the streets of midtown where he worked.

"God isn't ready for me," he said, looking straight at me, his eyes unwavering. "That's what I realized when I lost my lover, Ben, two years ago. I wanted him to take me too, or to have taken me instead of Ben. I loved Ben so very much, that's just the way I felt. But God didn't. So he wanted me to live, and live a good life, which is what I've tried to do. Maybe I'll be around for another forty years, just plugging away. There will be survivors in this epidemic, just as in war and in the Holocaust.

"Ben loved me. We were going to grow old together. It didn't happen, but I know that he's in heaven and I pray for him, and to him. He's still watching over me somehow. I believe that, because he was a good person and he loved me. I didn't want to lose him, and he didn't want to leave me. But his time was up.

"He left me all his possessions. We were married—as much a couple as any married people are. That's why I stayed with him when he got sick. He would have stayed with me.

"Now he's up there with God. I talk to him sometimes and ask him questions: What should I do, Ben? I know you're there. I feel your presence. He knows where I am and what's going on right now. He's happy and doesn't suffer anymore. I hear his voice, though not in a psychotic way. At times I wish I could, but I don't. His spirit is still watching over me though, guiding me. He yells at me sometimes, as he did in life. But he never yelled at me without love. You can't ask more than that. You can't.

"I've always been spiritual, but I'm more so now. I used to go to church once a week, but for the last two years I go at least three times a week. I'm Catholic and love the church I belong to. Mass is a beautiful thing to me. I pray to St. Jude—the Saint of Hopeless Causes. Even if I die of AIDS, I'm going to go to heaven, because I'll have tried. That's the important thing: you have to try. God has to know you're trying.

"In spite of what the Catholic church believes, I think God still loves me. I'm not going to lose my religion because of my sexuality. I was Catholic long before I became gay, even though I have felt gay since I was five years old. The church consists of man-made rules, but God made me this way. That doesn't exonerate me from any responsibility. But I hope the church will come around to realize that there are good gays. We're not all evil. Especially today.

"I don't know why God made us this way. To hold down the population? To channel our energies into other things? Frankly I don't consider myself a particularly creative person. I try to be creative in living: that's good enough for me.

"But I refuse to believe that HIV is going to get me. In a way, I've already beaten this thing. People said I should have had various symptoms. Well, I haven't, and many other people haven't either. Thank God.

"Other people bear their crosses. HIV is mine."

The Red Bags: New Beliefs

While Jason draws on earlier religious faith as a basis for his current beliefs, many patients after testing, now faced with the sudden threat of annihilation, undergo conversions and pursue spirituality for the first time.

Gregory Colson, the Vietnam veteran, grew up in a working-class neighborhood on Staten Island, the son of an alcoholic, and was involved in drugs from an early age. He is a wide-shouldered man with a black beard. When I first interviewed him he wore aviator glasses and kept his brown leather jacket on throughout. He sat firm, unmoving in his seat when he spoke. I would have been afraid to meet him on a dark street. He had used drugs, but not for several years. "My biggest fear is dying of the virus in jail," he told me, "because I've seen seven people pass away there from HIV and it's very lonely. Plus, I've been in jail half my life, and don't want to die there too.

"I got tested in prison in 1986. Joey, a friend of mine, told me that he and another friend of ours had the virus, and that I should take the test since we had shared needles. I took it, and two weeks later the nurse called me into her office and said I was positive. I asked her what that meant, and she said, 'You have AIDS. You have two to six months to live.' I was shocked. I cried. I had never cried before—not when my mother died, not when my girlfriend had cancer, not when we lost our child, not when I faced four life sentences. But HIV was the last straw.

"I wondered, would I survive to go to the parole board? Would somebody find out? There's so many prejudices and fears in prison. There's a list of grievances that will automatically get you stabbed, slashed, or killed . . . anyone considered nonhuman, un-acceptable—a snitch, an informer, a child abuser, or someone with AIDS. On the way back to my cell after getting my results, things I had seen a million times I now saw through different eyes, as if for the first time—the bars, the other men's faces.

"I didn't tell anybody except Joey. He used to run around the yard twenty times a day and was as big as a house. But a few months after I was tested, his nails started falling off, and he dete-riorated from 210 pounds to 130.

"One day I went to the hospital to visit him, and the nurse told me he had passed away. I couldn't believe it. I wanted something of his to remember him by. They had his belongings in a little sep-arate room in red bags, 'because,' the nurse told me, 'if anybody touches his clothes, they can catch it.' I had to put on gloves and a mask, and went in and took out a yellow sweatsuit, with a hood and pants, and washed them by hand.

"A few nights later I wore them into the yard. Some of my friends saw me and asked, 'Do you have AIDS?' I said, 'No.' And they said, 'Well, Joey had AIDS . . .' And I said, 'No, no, I got this from somebody else.' Then people came over and said, 'You know, people are getting firebombed here if it's known they have AIDS.' And I said, 'I don't have AIDS. I'm not gay, and only gay people get AIDS.' At that time prisons didn't have much information. People also figured they could get HIV from you if you used the shower and touched the hand bar, or got some of your body fluids on the soap, or sneezed.

"All of a sudden, though, I started getting very religious. I started really believing in God and the Bible. I wasn't religious when I was young. I was raised in the Pentecostal church. On Sundays my mother would drag me to church with her. I now said to God, 'Please, I don't want to die in jail.' All I wanted to do was to be able to die on the outside. I've done about seventeen years in prison, by the way, in and out all my life for drugs. All I kept thinking now was, damn, I'm going to die in jail! Didn't I do enough time here already?

"I went to church and prayed, and changed my life around. I said to God, 'You know that I've killed people, and didn't mean it. I'm not a killer. Basically I'm not a bad guy. I mean, I've done time in prison, but it certainly hasn't been because I've elected to be a criminal. I've been hurt, molested, abused, and raped. I never found a woman who loved me. My own mother and father didn't love me. Now I've got the virus. But please don't let me die here.' And something clicked in my head: 'If I let you go out, you're gonna kill people.' So I said, as if I were just talking to you now, 'Dear Lord, if you let me out, Lord, if you let me out, I'm not going to kill a soul.'

"I stopped hanging out with people that were using drugs. I got into a drug program, and they helped get me released. I wasn't supposed to get out this soon either.

"I'm not even supposed to be alive right now. I've had people looking to kill me because I robbed them. I don't snatch people's pocketbooks or steal their TVs. I rob people who won't call the cops because they're doing the same thing I am—selling drugs or being bookies or pimps. So I rationalized that it was okay. But it's not okay. Also, they didn't call the cops, but I've been stabbed four or five times, hit on the head with a pipe, and shot—twice in the leg and once in my finger. My life hasn't been a bowl of cherries. I've had to pay for the things I've done.

"I'm a survivor, though. I've been in riots in prison at Green-haven and Rikers Island. I was in jail when the Attica riot happened. Guys once put guns to both sides of my head and said they were going to kill me unless I got down on my knees and begged. And I wouldn't beg. I've been in car accidents in which people died. I was thrown out of a window in Harlem—three stories up. I've just had a very rough and violent life. I don't get anything easily.

"So I believe that God is up there looking over me, because I'm not supposed to be here today for the things I've done. I know people who didn't do nothing like I did, and got killed for it. I once saw a guy get killed for ten dollars. I've seen a person in jail get killed for a pair of sneakers. I overdosed seven or eight times and was declared dead once—in the hospital my heart stopped from a heroin overdose in 1968. I've been at death's door many times but didn't die.

"Why? It wasn't luck. God wants me here for a reason: to do good. He doesn't want me to die. He wants me to help other people, to be a messenger, and spread the word—about how to protect yourself from HIV, and how to live with it if you've already got it, and how not to give it to somebody else. I volunteer now, visiting AIDS wards almost every day, talking to patients no one else visits. Yesterday a girl asked me for a cigarette. I said, 'I'll give you two, but you have to do me a favor. Fix yourself. Your chest is all hanging out, that's not right.' She said, 'I thought you were a counselor, or from social service.' I said 'Why, because of my beard and glasses? I have the virus just like you. But I'm a man, and you're a woman. If I was laying in bed exposed and you came in, I hope you would tell me to cover myself. You have to respect yourself so other people will respect you.'

"If I didn't have the virus, I wouldn't be here or be as caring as I am today. I was very evil and very violent. And I tell a lot of people that I couldn't hurt anybody today. I believe that if you do good, good will come your way, and if you do bad, bad comes your way. I'm not a preacher or a crusader, but I believe now that good can overpower bad. When I was a drug addict I didn't do normal things. I wasn't normal. HIV has made me normal."

Although they come from different backgrounds, Jason and Gregory respond to HIV primarily by seeking spiritual answers and contexts for their despair. Spirituality comforts and reassures them that they are part of something larger and more ongoing than themselves.

Each man approaches and interprets religion in his own way. Gregory views the relationship in tangible and concrete terms. God helped him get out of jail, in turn he does God's work. Jason wants communication with his former boyfriend, the sense that the latter's death is neither a permanent nor definitive loss. Jason also accepts religion but separates himself from some of the church's practices and teachings.

Both men believe God intervenes in everyday life, mediating fate and the course of illness, thus reducing randomness and vulnerability. God determines whether and when they will die from the virus, and provides hope that the virus might not advance inside them.

These two men also believe that God does not punish but will help them if they try to help themselves. "I'm no saint," Jason added, as he considered past sexual encounters. But he has faith that God will nonetheless protect him. Both he and Gregory construct a religiosity that permits a few slipups. God's forgiveness and continued support can be elicited through effort.

These notions might be seen as convenient and self-serving, but these men take their faith very seriously, speak with passion and conviction, and act on their beliefs. Gregory visits patients daily. The possibility of death has motivated him to sustain compassion for the first time in his life. Jason attends church three times a week. These men believe fervently that their spirituality helps them.

Many HIV-infected people who feel "positive" about the illness and trace this feeling to messages disseminated by the AIDS movement, have in fact become more spiritual, often in traditional ways. Yet the politicized nature of the disease has compelled many to attribute their success in coping with the virus to more politically sanctioned statements about "living with HIV," even though religion has been critical, giving these men and women the sense that some part of their spirit will continue on. Political action in HIV-land is fundamentally antireligious, valuing political over other concerns. Religions are not rational, logical, or universally agreed on. Partly as a result, political reasons for accepting a positive HIV status are more socially sanctioned than spiritual ones, yet the two often operate together.

Choosing Churches

The issue is not only whether to be religious, but how—how to find a spiritual tradition with which one can feel connected. Many patients reject Western organized religion and pursue Eastern or other non-Western spiritual ideas, or nontraditional New Age philosophies and crystals. Individuals often mix and match spiritual traditions, integrating old familiar ideas with more recently acquired beliefs in order to find comfortable modes.

Many reject the churches in which they were raised. Yvette Bing, who invoked the image of apartheid, explained, "I tried becoming religious, but churches didn't work for me. The Catholic faith doesn't like condoms. The church will help you die but won't help you stay alive. I couldn't understand that. The Episcopalians and the Baptists don't like people who use drugs or have been in prison. They claim they love God, but they don't love you. The Muslim faith doesn't have that and gives a black person dignity. But if God made all people equal, why must the women sit behind the men? So right now I'm just a person who believes in something mightier than man. I've always believed in a higher power. At the age of five I remember just knowing inside of me, without ever hearing it, that something made the trees and put the sun up there. I've had numerous spiritual awakenings throughout my life. I didn't know what they were, but they happened—instances where I've prayed and had the feeling that something put my body in a praying position. I believe there is a supreme being. If there weren't, I wouldn't still be here. So I thank God for every day I haven't gotten worse."

Roy Gifford, retiring, born and raised on a farm, and having studied biology, said, "I believe in the Third Law of Thermodynamics. Energy can neither be created nor destroyed, it merely goes on in another form. After death I assume I'll be heading in another direction, one way or another. Friends who have died of AIDS are just continuing on in a different form. I assume there's something out there, but I don't get bogged down in any one religious system. I take a little bit from here and there. I have a Quaker background, my mother is Pennsylvania Dutch and Lutheran, my father was Methodist. I used to joke that I would be married Jewish and buried Druid. I just lump them all together as 'the God fetish.' It's hard for me to imagine a total discontinuation of consciousness. If I thought that was all there was, I would not have hesitated to terminate the experience, because I saw no point in continuing, it was so bad.

"So I conceive of a continuation of consciousness, but I have no concept of what that will be like. It sounds very metaphysical, Indian and irrational, and I'm otherwise a very rational person. But to me the idea of death being nothing is offensive.

"Still, it's not religious! It's based not on any kind of religious belief but on a need to feel this isn't all there is."

Mitchell Walters, the Caucasian injecting drug user, looks to pagan roots, antedating the Catholic church, as an alternative. "Pan is a great God to pray to or invoke. He's the dude—part goat—that ran around chasing nymphets through the forest, drinking wine. In the Greek religion he is the god of merriment, sex, and partying. Christians tell you Pan is evil, the devil. But whatever I want to believe is my thing, and anyone who tells me I'm wrong and they're right is wrong.

"I go to church once, maybe twice a year. But I pray and talk to higher powers and spirits at least once a day. I have an altar at my house. An altar has to have the four elements that make up everything—air, water, fire, and earth. I have a wand that represents air, a candle, crystals, and a brass statue of the Pan. I bought the altar when I became HIV."

Afterlives: The Components of Religious Feeling

Within the spiritual worlds they construct for themselves, individuals adopt different sets of beliefs. Some, like Wilma, describe being "born again" since testing. As she says, "I was standing up on a mountaintop at an upstate retreat overlooking the Hudson River when all of a sudden I heard God's voice." Yet she traces this event not to her illness but to God directly, and denies that this experience resulted in any way from her being infected. "I feel like I just cleansed my soul out and have a new one now."

Beliefs about reincarnation are frequent. These notions vary from traditional religious views of the afterlife to a vague sense that "all this can't go completely to waste." Jason Gillian does not believe in reincarnation *per se* but in his lover continuing on and communicating from heaven. The spiritual enlightenment that many attain after infection allows them to connect their lives—the ends of which are now in sight—with a past and a future.

Alfie Montoya, who saw the virus as "slick," told me, "This is hell because you suffer here and go through a lot of pain. HIV is something you go through in hell. The way they punish you is to come back like this—being a bum or homeless. One day it's ninety-five degrees outside—fucking hot. The next day it's below zero. That's punishment. That's hell. Maybe I was real bad in a former life and am paying for it now. I believe in God a hundred percent, but in the devil too. Something makes you do good things, but something makes me do bad things, like going to drugs. Drugs are the evilest things around. The devil puts thoughts in my head: go do a bag, it won't hurt, nobody will know. Maybe the devil put HIV here. God wouldn't have. HIV gets rid of the junkies and homos. But what about the kids? They're not junkies or homos. God wouldn't be killing little kids. So it has to be the devil spreading AIDS. When God created human beings, there was no pain or hurt in the world. But Adam and Eve disobeyed him, and God said, 'For disrespecting me, you leave me no choice. I was preventing you from even getting there, but it seems you want to try this. Here it is.' The devil was one of God's most beautiful angels and wanted to sit with God, and God expelled him from on high to down here. Since he was the first one down here, he's the owner of all this. We have to pay for what Adam and Eve did. Once we leave here we go back up to him, to heaven, where there's no suffering and you have no needs. We're sure not going to go through what we go through now.

"I don't believe anybody stays here. We're going to live again with Christ. There'll be no more fighting, famines, or disease. It'll be a perfect world, without HIV or anything else to catch. That's something to look forward to."

Alfie and others also believe that the biblical Book of Revelations predicts the epidemic. "The Book of Revelations says there will be a scourge as part of the Apocalypse: there will be a last day, kids will rise up against their parents, mother against daughter. We won't be able to tell the seasons, there will be a war, nations will rise up against nations, there will be a plague with no cure. To me AIDS is the plague, affecting everybody all over the world. It's wiping out a whole generation. I hear such and such a person is dead: this one, that one's dead. My nephew and his girlfriend both just died of AIDS. A lot of things in Revelations are happening now. It says the world is going to be destroyed by fire. All these nuclear weapons are going to blow up and create a big fire. I believe it: the wars, and the rumors of wars, the fighting and disrespect. Instead of sitting down and talking and trying to find a solution, people just drop bombs and kill. Something incurable passes from person to person. My sense is that the world's going to come to an end pretty soon. Time's getting short. The things the Bible predicts will come true." HIV thus marks, in part, the end of the whole world, not just Alfie's life. He sees himself not as a lone victim of chance or chaos but as part of a larger, preordained plan. In an epidemic, social and individual experiences blur.

Second Chances: The Functions of Spirituality

Spirituality can serve many functions. A higher power can assuage regrets about one's life. As Eddie Lourdes said, "The only thing that's hell now is thinking of all the things I should have done but didn't—things I had and lost due to drugs. I'm sorry about what I've done and what I could have done. But there's nothing I can do about it now. And I did it to myself. I look back at my life a little more now. I don't like looking back at it too much because I get down. I know I messed up my life. I think about it so I don't make any mistakes, but I can't linger on it too much or I get down in a slump. I don't like my past, the things I did, so I don't like thinking about them. I get blue: I can't look forward to many things. Why the hell did this happen to me? I'm like Old Man River: tired of living and afraid of dying.

"But I lived my life the way I wanted to. It may not have been the best for other people, but it's how I lived it. If I wanted something, I'd use any means to get it: conning, conniving. If I talked to a person long enough, I could get anything I wanted from him. I didn't ask nobody for anything. In return, they didn't ask me for nothing. I didn't want to be obligated to anyone because people could use you that way. I used to pride myself on that. But now I realize that it ain't nothing to pride myself on. In my neighborhood they talk about me like a dog. I hurt a lot of people, I know, and if I could go back and change it all, I would. I'd do it totally different. But I can't do that now, and I have to accept that. I'm not proud of it, but I try to laugh about it since there's nothing else I can do.

"I did enough wrong for everybody in the family—everything that was out there to do. I was always in the middle of the gang. I could have been dead or in jail now. I thank God that I'm still sitting here. Only three or four people I grew up with are still here. The rest are all dead or in jail. I feel ashamed that I shot drugs and jumped into bed with any woman. I don't feel ashamed that I got HIV but about how I got it.

"In the end, though, we're all in God's hands. My mother says God has let me know I'm going to die. He has given me a second chance to come to him, to bring myself more to him. He gave me another chance, an opportunity, time to get myself prepared. God helps me. That's the bottom line. God has a purpose for everything, a master plan. He shakes you over the pit but doesn't let you fall. I can't blow it now. I try to take the negative and turn it around into a positive to keep my sanity. Life is like an electrocardiogram: it has ups and downs, but if it's done, you're dead. So when I have those bad days, I say a little prayer and try to turn things around and think of something positive that will outweigh the negative. The only things that help are spiritual beliefs.

"I have good days and bad days. A third of my days are still bad. That's the devil poking at me. He'll try to get me any way he can to make me feel down. He comes at me in all kinds of disguises. If I want to drink booze or shoot drugs, that's the devil, whom I try to avoid by staying clean." The term *clean* suggests not only being drug-free but also a moral position. Cleanliness is both physical and psychic.

Spirituality has other psychological consequences: it diminishes expectations, focuses attention on the here and now, and leads to a reordering of priorities as earlier pursuits become less important. Olana Ramirez, who had feared disintegration, says, "I've learned—not only because of the virus but because of my life experiences—not to look too far ahead. Even before HIV, a lot of plans I made in my life just fell apart. So I try to live more today and focus on what I can accomplish today. I don't know what tomorrow holds. I've seen people die every day without HIV. Nobody has a guarantee. So I'm going to live every day to its fullest and enjoy every minute I can. When the bad times come, I'll fight them. I don't know if I'll be here tomorrow. I can go out and get hit by a car. All of us have our dates set, with or without HIV, so I look at it as if I didn't have the virus. It's whenever God wants me." Thus she can achieve a feeling of wholeness, at least in the moment.

Many believe spirituality can heal them. Matt Winchell sees spiritual beliefs as capable of improving his health. Herbal holistic medicine enables him to feel he can exercise more control over his fate and reduce his helplessness. He closely follows the writings of Louise Hay, who has written self-help books and recorded popular audiotapes on holistic health and self-healing, and Bernie Siegel, who describes (as in *Love, Medicine and Miracles*) the power of the mind to heal the body. The lack of full scientific support for such beliefs does not deter Matt, for he views the medical profession skeptically, as self-serving. Primarily he trusts that belief can heal his body and reverse undesired biological processes.

Others have difficulty connecting religion to physical or psychological healing. Jenny Singer said, "I have gone to Louise Hay seminars and try to follow her book. It helps very much, but I'm not consistent with it. Some of the exercises are hard, especially when I have to look into a mirror and tell me how much I like myself. I find that difficult because I don't always like myself, and I'm angry at myself a lot. Louise Hay advises changing the way I think: I should never say 'I should have,' or put myself down for things. But it's very hard. I'm religious, not with an organized religion but with me personally. I don't go to church but I pray to God. My husband and I also read the Bible every day and talk about it. It's a kind of combined religion. I was born Jewish and still believe in Judaism, but I also believe in Jesus Christ. Reverend Butterworth preaches the power of positive belief—believing in yourself and in the Lord and loving one another. It's not any kind of organized religion by itself, just a general thing.

"I never used to pray every day. But when I get up now I pray for being alive and being able to see a new day. I'm much more grateful for being able to walk and for the basic things in life. But I'm still very frightened of dying. I think a lot about what's on the other side. I never used to give heaven and hell much thought, but now I'm wondering if there really are such places."

Without Faith

Yet not all who seek religious reassurance find it. A lack of faith may be the consequence of numerous factors, including unsatisfying earlier experiences with religion. Robert Banoff, a young gay man, said, "I am not at all a spiritual person. I would like to be, but I don't understand how." He sports a crew cut and an earring and wears a black leather jacket with metal snaps and buckles. "When I grew up, my parents belonged to an Orthodox synagogue. They took me but were not at all religious. For them Judaism was more cultural than spiritual. They went because they had always gone, and everyone they knew went. But I need to understand things and to have something tangible. Religion doesn't do that for me. If there really is a God, why is he so cruel? Why are people suffering? ACT-UP gives me concrete results. Religion doesn't."

A few have lost their religion as a result of HIV, as many did because of the Holocaust. Aaron Eliot said, "I'm of the Jewish faith but not a practicing Jew. I just lost faith. There is too much agony in this world. So much suffering of innocent people. I engaged in high-risk activity, though we didn't know it at the time. But all these innocent people around the world, starving. Why? Is there a reason? Is there really a God above? I've become very skeptical and cynical about it. I lost faith after finding out I was HIV positive. I became much more aware of all the suffering around the world. If you are not there, you don't see it—except on television and you say, 'Oh, how awful,' and turn it off. But when you are sick, the suffering has more meaning.

"A friend of mine is very spiritual, which I admire greatly. I wish I had some, that it would rub off on me. But it just doesn't. It never happened. I'm not that type of person."

Maurice Bradford too says, "I wish I could believe in God, but I can't seem to. Occasionally I go to church, but more because my partner used to go before he died than because I believe.

"I pray in my own way. I wish this and that. I don't ask for forgiveness, because I have no regrets. I am what I am. Certain things I could have done better, but what the hell? Here I am. I feel like a hypocrite because for forty-eight years I haven't prayed and all of a sudden now I believe? I still don't believe. It's not only that I wasn't practicing. I don't believe. Or, prove it to me, it's not enough that the world exists. Anyway, proof isn't forthcoming, at least not yet."

Religious orthodoxies and institutions repel many, particularly in this age of skepticism toward authoritative institutions. Leonard Barber, in Westchester, avoids HIV-land. "I have a massive aversion to anything remotely twelve-step," he says, "because of the religious over-, under-, and through-tones of much of what they do. I'm insulted if I'm told to subordinate my being, intellect, and personality to some so-called higher power." He lives away from the center of HIV-land and works as a gardener, focusing on nature as revealing the hand of God in an almost pagan way.

Many remain agnostic. George Sullivan said, "I thought I might have squeaked through, that due to the complete absurdity of the universe I would manage to get away with it." Overall most people see the universe as ordered, not as chaotic or absurd. Yet grey areas clearly exist between belief and doubt.

Those without some form of spirituality tend to be more depressed, though it is difficult to know which came first—their inability to recognize a spiritual dimension to their lives or their broader despair.

Why Me?

HIV prompts many patients to see the universe as a moral place in which they try to place themselves. Spirituality can involve a search to make sense of behavior seen by oneself or others as immoral. As a result, patients often come to view the virus as both a punishment and an opportunity for redemption.

As suggested earlier, some see HIV as retribution from God. Lorraina Ortiz, who had to eat from paper plates at her mother's house, said, "Sometimes I go into a pity pile and ask, 'Why me?' Then I say, 'Well, I deserve it.' I have a lot of guilt about a lot of things, because I did so many things. I feel guilty about my prostitution. I try to justify why I did it: I had an addiction. Yet in my upbringing, prostitution was condemned. Still, I stooped that low to do it. I also have a lot of guilt about my children. There were times in their lives when I wasn't home and should have been. I was 'out there.' I always had custody but walked away from the responsibility. I left my husband and kids and just went out on my own. The longest period was for three years. I came back only after my husband went out looking for me. A cousin of mine had called him and said, 'Please help her out, she needs help.' I was right there in the Bronx but out on the street, drugging during the night and living in abandoned buildings during the day. I was already coming down with a lot of diseases. So sometimes I think HIV is a punishment for all the wrong things I did: dealing with drugs, robbing, stealing from my parents when they tried to be good to me. That's why I got the virus, because a lot of things I did were wrong. I used to shoplift and got away with a lot of stuff that didn't belong to me. I did a lot of damage at home, stealing radios in the house and money out of my mother's purse. And these things are not right. Maybe in some way God gave me the virus— put it back to me. I don't think like that all the time, but to a certain degree. You reap what you sow." Lorraina's universe remains balanced and equitable, even if unforgiving.

She tries to reframe her life positively in this moral context but still meets difficulties. "I do have a few regrets, I hate to say, because I wasted a lot of time in my life. I had a lot of opportunities to do things, and didn't. But today, as long as I try to stay clean and do the right thing, I'll be okay. I have to consider myself grateful for some of those experiences in the past. They happened for a reason, I guess. Sometimes you have to suffer before something good comes out of it.

"So I want to think positive and do right, but part of me is out of my control. It's like two different lives. Part of me is in control, part of me is not.

"At the clinic the staff always has trouble finding a vein for taking blood from me. They have to use my neck. Every time they poke me with a needle, I feel I'm being punished, that I did this to myself by abusing drugs. Blood drawing normally takes five minutes. Mine can last an hour." Unfortunately she can't fully reconcile or combine the parts of her life, and continues to use drugs.

Many patients whom I treated with psychotherapy in the HIV mental health clinic in New York City, who felt "punished" for their "sins," often resisted change. They felt these beliefs resulted from religion, not psychological states. That sex, the source of life, can now also cause death, reinforces Christian morality with its strong sanctions against activities that transmit the virus.

Many wrestle with this issue of whether they "deserve" the illness. Wilma Smith, for instance, changes her stance on this issue over time. "At first I tried to say I didn't deserve this virus," she reported. "I thought I wasn't promiscuous. But at the rehab, when I had to write down all my past sexual partners in black and white, I thought, 'Come on, Wilma, you've got a list down to the bottom of the page and you're still writing.' Then I felt really ashamed. I had to make the list era by era because that's the only way I could.

Names kept popping up. What about so-and-so? Oh yeah, I forgot about him. Being HIV positive, I'm lucky that's all I am. I'm lucky I don't try to get up in the morning and the waist down remains in the bed and the waist up walks away.

"All the drugs, and going to bed with men I would not ordinarily have gone with—it was just a vicious cycle. I'd be under the influence, or have an ulterior motive: my rent was due. I didn't stand on a corner and sell my body, but basically it was the same shit. It was not a one-night stand—that's what made it different. It was 'a relationship.' But it was really the same thing, because if you took away the money, then forget it, Buster—you know, one of those kinds of deals. I mean, God, where was my self-respect? Where were my values? All the while I had these things but hardly stayed dressed enough to realize it. I was always in somebody's bed for one reason or other. But that's just not Wilma, that's not the behavior I'm proud of." She tries to separate herself from this culpable behavior.

"The pain of that, and the fact I was positive made me afraid of having to call these men and tell them. But the rehab told me I was endangering their lives by not telling them. The things the rehab told me! When I came back to New York, I found out it didn't have to be done that way. But I wasn't yet back in New York. I was in Georgia and had to abide by their rules and regulations. So I got on the phone and called as many of these men as I could, with the exception of a few I couldn't contact. Some were supportive and told me to take care and not to worry, and they would pray for me. But others called me a bitch, a whore—everything but a child of God—and I clung to these negative things."

Gregory Colson, after becoming religious in prison, saw HIV not as punishment but as a symbolic message, "a warning from God: his way of telling me to pull my life together." Gregory thus changed his behavior by stopping drugs and volunteering, trying to achieve redemption.

Jason rejects church teachings, believing God will forgive and understand him, even if the church won't. He also subscribes to an overriding system of moral justice. "One physician cut Ben's lung in a test for PCP," he said. "That doctor will burn in hell as far as I'm concerned. He'll get his. I know. It happens to me: if I wrong someone, it comes back to haunt me."

Others disagree that HIV has anything to do with Providence. Yvette Bing, who didn't pick up her test results, said, "I don't think I deserve this. God is supposed to be loving and good. Why would he give somebody something that sucks? I believe it's something that just happens. It just so happened that at the time I was involved in drugs, HIV was going around. Through my own irresponsibility, I happened to get it. I don't ask God for anything except to give me strength to do what I have to do, or to keep my kids strong. When I pray, I'm only asking God to keep me from getting an ego and gaining false pride. God only helps those who help themselves. It only works if you work it. I work with him, and he works with me." Her relationship with God sounds businesslike, involving a give and take, like the world of drugs. Nonetheless she believes it is up to her to initiate and maintain changes in her life.

Given the suffering they experience and the innocence they feel, many individuals, searching for a moral explanation, seek to assign responsibility. This concern becomes prominent for them. Carrie Serano, a Latina former injecting drug user, in order to overcome her sense of responsibility, tries to blame others and redeem herself. She said, "My second husband was in jail, and it kept bothering me that we used to share needles. I asked him if he had taken the test, and he said he had in jail, and that it had come out negative. But for some reason it kept bothering me. So when he came out of jail, I told him I wanted us to get tested. He refused the first couple of times but eventually gave in. When the results came back, my inner me knew I was going to be positive.

"It was hard. I thought of my kids. I wasn't going to have much time for them; I was gonna die. What was I gonna do? I thought of the mistake I had made in using drugs anyway. Thank God for some reason I had already stopped.

"I had started shooting drugs only after I was married, and only for a year. My husband has been on them for God knows how long—since he was growing up. I didn't know how to face him. I didn't want to tell him, 'It's your fault,' because I didn't really know. But when I found out our T-cell counts, something told me he gave it to me because my T-cell count was over a thousand while he needed AZT. I wanted to tell him then, 'It's your fault. It's not because I did this to myself.'

"I often think, 'Why me? Of all people, why me?' If I didn't have HIV I would probably live longer. But then I think, God, I'm not dying. If I take care of myself I'll be here for a while. Maybe I'll live what I'm supposed to live even though I have the virus."

"Other times I get scared. I did drugs for such a short time. I don't know how to explain it. I condemn myself for using drugs. But I look at the reasons why I did it. My first husband hung himself, and I felt guilty about it. It's no excuse, but I was in the wrong place at the wrong time: drugs were there and I used them. They were the only escape I had. I was alone. My husband was a heavy drinker. He didn't abuse me, though sometimes I wish he *had* hit me rather than tell me the things he used to. Sometimes you can hurt a person verbally more than physically. He would also come home drunk and use our credit card to go to motels with other women. I got venereal diseases like they were going out of style." Carrie thus sees herself as a victim, not fully responsible.

"I also didn't want our children to have a stepfather or be raised without a dad. But meanwhile they were going through this, seeing me cry all the time. I had had about ten stepfathers, and they used to hit my mother, who was a registered nurse, dislocating her arms and breaking her ribs. That always stayed in the back of my mind. I didn't want to give my kids that example. But meanwhile I was giving them the example of drugs. Jesus! So my husband and I finally separated. Four months later he killed himself. That really blew my mind. His family blamed me. His brother would call me at night, and say, 'Murderer,' and hang up. That played with my head. Finally I said, 'You know what's bothering you? Your conscience. You killed your brother.' He never called again after that, but that's when I started doing drugs. That's when my life went downhill.

"The worst drug is crack. That was my downfall. I started it when my brother took my son and my daughter got pregnant. My whole life cracked. I had no scruples, values, or goals. Everything was that damn drug. Still, I never neglected my little one. She always ate something before she went to bed, and went to school. And I never went to jail. But I did neglect her by hardly being with her. I would lock myself in my room, get high, and forget she was even there. She would knock on the door, and say, 'Mommy,' and I would tell her, 'Later, leave me alone.' I didn't think about my kids—I didn't think about anything. But that's not me. I'm a very devoted mother, and the crack just took that from me." Carrie splits off a good, responsible self from a bad, substance-abusing self, and attributes her problems to her husband's death, his family, and drugs.

"At first I thought HIV was my punishment for being stupid enough to use drugs and share needles. I shouldn't have done what I did. But now I think this was just meant to happen. I know I made mistakes, but I still don't deserve to have HIV. I haven't been such a bad person. I try to help everybody. The other day, walking in the street, I saw a dirty drunk guy lying there and I gave him a sandwich I had in my hand. I was once out in the street and know the deal. I'll give something to eat but not money to get high. Now we also go out a lot with our baby—she's eight, but we call her the baby—to the zoo, to the park. We try to give her what we didn't when we were getting high. We were like cats and dogs. But not now. We try to make it up to her. It can never be replaced because it happened, but we try.

"Maybe there is a higher meaning to what I'm going through. I try to look at it as positive. Maybe this is what's been written in The Big Book for me to go through. I think God is testing me. I have to prove myself, like Job."

Issues concerning fate arise commonly. Questions of 'Why me?', asked by Carrie and others, refer on one hand to mechanics and the probability of transmission, and on the other hand to moral justification. Yet the two sets of meanings blur.

HIV as fate provides a sense of coherence and completion. Roger Babson, the gay man living in an AIDS residence, said, "After my diagnosis, I thought about the wonderful things and the bad things that happened in my life. I pulled out two pieces of paper, one to list the terrible things—the alcohol, the homelessness, living in the shelter, having AIDS. On the other sheet I was going to list the good things—going sailing with the Kennedys once, and knowing the friends and wonderful people in my life. Then I realized this should all be the same piece of paper—the good and the bad—because they're all life's experiences. I came to this great realization that everything is a blessing, what was intended for me. So I saw it in a positive way. I didn't feel like I was being punished, but I felt this was part of my destiny. Had I not been diagnosed, I might have been a little bit more callous." Thus he is able to integrate desired and undesired aspects of his life, and see death as part of a whole. Destiny is not only foretold but final and all-encompassing. The notion of a predetermined plan prevails.

Fate can also reflect not divine or supernatural intervention but inevitability, an extension of the life heretofore led. Jill Montgomery, who now tries to surround herself with positive people, said, "HIV is a total breakdown of body functioning. The way I lived, there was no recourse but for me to have a breakdown in my body's communication and protection. Drugs have given me countless staph infections and done an up-and-down pendulum job on my body metabolism—no sleeping, no eating. Through twenty-three years of drug abuse I've been hospitalized for various infections, and it stands to reason that after these things take their toll, there is nowhere else to go. What happened was simply inevitable. They say the virus was made to destroy a sect of people. All I know is that after the constant bombardment, month after month, year after year, the constant tearing down from infectious diseases, my immune system really had no choice but to go crazy. Had I not stopped drugs, I'd be dead. I didn't have no respect or appreciation for nobody telling me nothing, because of my drug addiction and lifestyle. It was all about 'get yours.' I've been medicated all my life. The way I look at it, ever since I can remember I've had some form of this virus. Now I can't stop it. It's there, written. There is no return. I don't believe they can make or give me anything that will restore the damage that's already been done.

"Eventually, if I don't get shot or hit by a bus, the virus will take me out. It's only a matter of time. Anybody in exactly my condition would have come to the same thing."

Such fatalism can fuel continued drug use or unsafe sex. "Once a doctor asked me how long I had been using drugs, and I told him twenty-three years. He said, 'You know, it's time for you to stop.' I knew, but didn't know how. How could I live without a drug? He told me I was going to die soon. I said, he's crazy. I thought God wasn't going to take me out the way he was telling me."

Others feel HIV is inevitable though still not deserved. Alfie Montoya said, "I could have the attitude: why the fuck did you let me get HIV? But then again, how the fuck could I not get it with all the things I did, the needles I used. I actually used water from a goddam toilet bowl one time. I figured, well, I'm shooting it in the cap, heating it up in the flame and boiling it, so it'll be all right.

There was no water anywhere else and I had to do it right away. It was a bathroom and people were knocking on the door. I wanted to get it done with, so I took the water, put it in the cap, and boiled it. But using water from a toilet bowl is sick. I was tempting fate. So sometimes I've been stupid. But I still don't think I deserve to be HIV. Nobody does. When I started shooting drugs, I didn't know about it. If I did, I would still have done heroin but wouldn't have shot it. I'd snort it and also get better dope." Even with HIV, he refuses to censure his own drug use.

Raoul Rodriquez, the gay man from Mexico, remains uncertain, struggling to understand his role, blaming God but then himself, and looking to God for help. "I cry and am angry about life and say why? I never had an opportunity. I blame God for AIDS. I say, 'God, you know that I'm a good person. You understand me. I haven't hurt anybody, yet all my life I've suffered, trying to accept myself. God, why didn't you give me the opportunity to be happy? All my life has been a fight.' We Catholics pray to our Father, and one part is very significant for me: Come to earth. Please, God, take control of things. Take me over. I feel alone, overwhelmed by life. Show me the way. Don't leave me alone. Take my life if you want, but show me how I should live it. Catholicism says God created us and set us free, and we later get punished based on whether we have behaved or not. But so many things are out of my control. I get overwhelmed and say, 'Don't let me be free, I can't control my life.'" Raoul looks to God to compensate for his own sense of weakness, stemming in part from his low self-esteem.

Yet he remains conflicted. "Sometimes I have my religious doubts. Deep inside I believe. I want to believe. I pray every day. But sometimes I have difficulty imagining God. If he really exists, why did he let all these things happen?" Raoul's questions resemble those of many Holocaust survivors.

In the end he faults himself. "Sometimes I feel this disease is punishment for not having moral control. I don't give more weight to homosexuality than I do to any other sin. Everybody has sins. It's something I have to work with constantly, but I don't think God hates me because of that. He doesn't hate. I think of homosexuality as a sin because the Bible tells me it is. I accept it as part of my sinful nature, and I accept that all mankind has a sinful nature. But it was my fault I got HIV. Not for being gay, but just for not being really moral. Using drugs is immoral, having sex without being married is immoral, having homosexual encounters is immoral."

Raoul has had difficulty accepting his homosexuality and HIV infection, in part because he has seen gay friends in Mexico attacked, stoned by crowds in the street. "I just want to die happy with myself," he now says. "As happy as I can be. I feel let down by this fucking life, but I'm fighting back. I've gone from being passive to active. I'm still miles away from where I want to be, but at least I'm working on my self-esteem. AIDS has given me the strength to try.

"When I first found out I had AIDS, I prayed to God not to have a painful death. Now I pray for a peaceful rest of life. It doesn't matter if it's one month or three. I just want to die without regretting having lived."

Maurice Bradford, an atheist, faults himself without invoking God, but also becomes depressed. "I was bright enough to know early on that something risky was going on. I should have stopped my avoidance and denial and tried to modify my behavior more successfully. But I don't think I'm being punished. It was just stupidity, or maybe a little weakness, but nothing more than that. Once in a while I wonder, 'Why me?' and I say, 'Me, because I fucked around without protection.' But it's possible I contracted this virus before anybody even knew it existed. I can't blame myself."

Overall few see God as punishing. Lorraina Ortiz, rejected by her family, still uses drugs and is one of the few participants who did not appear for a second interview. Raoul debates, first blaming God but then himself, and asking God for strength. A simplistic view of divine justice, of punishment and reward—an eye for an eye, a tooth for a tooth—arises from the Bible. Proverbs 12:21, for example, says, "No ills befall the righteous, but the wicked are filled with trouble." Yet to view God as punishing rather than solacing is painful. In such a universe the individual cannot win and has less room for hope. Those who are depressed may feel this way regardless. But most individuals believe in a cosmos in which hope is possible, in which God is ultimately forgiving, does not automatically or unilaterally punish, and takes into account extenuating or remitting circumstances.

Howard Kushner, in *When Bad Things Happen to Good People*, advocates that people accept randomness in the universe and look to God for strength. But few HIV-infected men and women talked of randomness. Most acknowledged their own contribution to their infection, even if mechanical. Complete randomness is difficult to tolerate, leading to resignation and sadness, and seeming to cancel out the existence of a God. These men and women rarely felt in the end that God held them responsible. They saw him as providing strength, particularly if they tried to gain his grace.

To achieve a further sense of innocence, as well as to focus anger, many attribute their infection to particular sexual partners. Wilma, for example, though initially feeling guilty, later pointed to one man whom she thought infected her. "I just needed to know who I contracted it from. I found out that one man in my past was an IV drug user. My doctor explained that didn't necessarily mean he was the one, but I went through the incubation period in my mind, and it had to be him, it had to be.

"I let go of the anger through psychotherapy. I pretended he was in a chair and I told him all the things I wanted to, releasing what I was feeling, which was a lot.

"Then two years later I saw this individual in the supermarket. I had always said that if I saw him, I'd spit in his eye, I'd do this, I'd do that, without any real evidence that he was the one who gave it to me. But I felt so strongly it was him.

"So seeing him in the supermarket I now had a chance to vent all this. And I said, 'Hey.' And he said, 'What's up, kid?' And that was it. End of conversation. I went down to the end of the aisle. Then the anger hit me. It was a delayed reaction. Had I not gone to psychotherapy, I would have been a madwoman and run up to him, scratching and clawing. By the time I got to the end of the aisle I *was* angry, because he was also one of the ones who didn't support me when I had called him up from Georgia. He told me that because he used intravenously, he always went to get tested. To this day I still don't know whether he's positive. But he was the only one in my past who I knew used IV drugs, and I'm not ready to let go of that theory yet. Anyway, at the supermarket I went back to look for him but he was gone. Maybe he just forgot something and had to run out, but it seems like he disappeared too quickly."

Wilma's belief that one man is responsible also enables her to channel her rage. She also seeks to assuage her own guilt for having decided to sleep with him while under the influence of alcohol and cocaine.

Women, more than gay men, blame other individuals. Many gay men have had more partners who could have infected them, and those gay men who do attribute their disease to a particular individual have had fewer partners. Roy Gifford, who had slept with only a handful of men in his life, said, "I know Tom infected me. After we were involved, he told me he had once been a call boy." Although it isn't clear that Tom is the one who in fact exposed him, Roy nonetheless tries to target his anger and frustration, and reduce the uncertainty involved.

As noted earlier, the HIV community discourages thinking of oneself as a victim and instead urges "empowerment." While this notion is politically sanctioned and perhaps even psychologically beneficial, many nonetheless find it easier to discuss than to achieve. Nor is the term's meaning always clear.

HIV-land also channels blame away from the self and onto "the system," with many accusing the government of instigating the epidemic or of not doing enough to halt it. Individual doctors get blamed for being ignorant or callous. Yet self-blame also persists. The political force of HIV-land does not wholly erase a psychological tendency to adopt a moral perspective and experience guilt. For good or bad, people view their lives and illnesses in moral terms—a human trait that must be understood and not just dismissed as incorrect.

This moral outlook reduces randomness. As among the Fore in Papua New Guinea, a system—even if flimsy or flawed—that can explain the disaster provides order. A higher principle, not mere chaos, prevails. The need to feel that the world is coherent becomes acute when a prior sense of wholeness has shattered.

Flowers and Fruits: Connections to Nature

Many of those with HIV seek to connect to nature as a way of sensing the implicit hand of God. Nature offers consolation and larger order. Leonard Barber in Westchester reported, "For the last three years I've been involved in a garden design business. The therapeutic aspects of gardening are clear: simply doing, being active. Though gardening design is very long term, the actual practice of horticulture is very immediate, with concrete physical progress that's very helpful. If my task is deadheading five thousand irises, I just do the job and it's done, which is very satisfying. In the meantime my mind can go off and think about anything it wants.

"Gardening is also useful in thinking about HIV because making and keeping a garden is about orchestrating death and dying. All plants have a life span. Annuals are purely seasonal, but perennials die at different rates. So making a garden is all about coordinating life: blooming, flowering, and fruiting. I have to understand how and when plants die and what to do to make sure the garden as a whole continues. I've got to accommodate all that dying. There's constantly going to be dying. I have to think in terms of decades. If I start a garden of any size this spring, it will be at least five years before I know what mistakes I make now. I might die before it does. To work with big trees, whose life spans are hundreds of years, I already have to project myself into a world in which I no longer exist. So I've developed a certain detachment from the results of my actions. If I can detach myself enough, I don't care that I'm doing something that won't come into its own until forty or fifty years after I'm gone. It's really just a matter of scale. If I die in five years, I don't get to see what I would have in twenty."

Nature can provide evidence of a higher power. Olana Ramirez said, "Yesterday evening I looked at the sky. It was a beautiful sunset, orange and purple. When I look at something like that, I know there's got to be something greater to create so much beauty out there. Man can't create that. So I have a lot of faith in a higher power. It's blind faith, but it beats no faith at all.

"Now I pray every night. I say, 'God.' The first part I say in Spanish because that's the way I learned it when I was in church. I'll start talking like I was talking to a person. Sometimes I ask him to forgive me for being weak. In a way I'm glad I'm HIV positive because it has made me see and appreciate a lot of things. I never noticed when it was going to rain, or the sky was beautiful, or the evening when the sun goes down. I thought drugs were it. I didn't need anything else."

Olana also sees evidence in biological processes of God and life continuing after death. "What fascinates me is how the body is built. I've seen videotapes about the immune system fighting, and it's beautiful. I feel joy when I see it. God made us perfect. He made one little cell to send a message and another cell to go fight, and they communicate to one another. The eyes see, and the liver filters things out. When I think of things like that, I'm grateful we have the ability to fight. Scientifically it's incredible. Would God create something so magnificent just to live a little while and die and be buried and that's it? There has to be something else. I'm put here for a purpose. God has something else planned for me. I don't know what.

"I don't believe I'll come back as a bird or nothing. But I always had the sense that this is just one part of my life. Nobody builds anything so beautiful, so intricate, and just throws it away. That's ridiculous."

Nature provides a sense of order in the face of chaos. Roy Gifford: "When I got totally frustrated the other week, I tore my fish tank apart and redid it. I couldn't move furniture around. My roommate walked in late in the evening and said, 'You must have been upset because you rearranged the fish tank.' I took everything out—all the stones and stuff—and relandscaped. I felt, 'There: life is reordered.' I don't have access to my other old ways of feeling balanced. In the past, when I had a car, I would drive to certain places, like up a hill, and just sit and look at the river. Or I'd go to a spring. I had favorite places. I still take walks, to no specific place. Just wherever the spirit goes. I forget about whatever upsets me, leave it behind or work it through."

Nature provides a sense of connection to the hereafter. As Jenny Singer said, "When a person knows they're going to die, they appreciate nature. I look at the clouds and the birds more. I go sit out on the porch at night and look up at the stars, and think, 'This is beautiful—the human body, the stars, and the leaves.' Nothing dies in this world. A tree loses its leaves, but they go on to become something else. Everything is part of a cycle. A supreme being definitely put all this together. I look up and see the sky and feel I want to be there one day. I didn't even think about death before HIV."

Nature serves as an escape. Jenny added, "Sometimes I just walk down by the river from 200th Street down to 125th Street, and simply keep walking. Wherever, whatever, it doesn't matter. The water comforts and calms me. I look at the sky just to put my mind in a state that I forget everything until I have to go back home. I also like the sound of water running. At home I turn on the faucet and just sit and let the water go through my hand, listening, like when it rains."

Spirituality can reduce the threat of death and alleviate feelings of rejection and isolation by making one feel accepted by God and an integral part of the larger, ongoing universe. Thus spirituality counters the threat of physical death and present and future social annihilation. Beliefs in a higher power serve other functions as well, providing a sense of order and an increased appreciation of the present. Individuals choose spiritual beliefs from a range of traditions and incorporate a variety of notions about communication with God—afterlife, Apocalypse, and physical healing. Nature too can provide order, escape, and evidence of God's existence. Yet not all who seek spiritual solace through these means find it, due in part to feelings of depression and past experiences with religion.

Issues of responsibility also press forcefully through these narratives. Given their earlier moral and religious beliefs, these individuals have a strong need to feel innocent. Most come to see God not as punishing but as forgiving and providing strength. Spirituality also assuages guilt about the past. Those who don't view HIV as God's will often see it as fate—if not a moral judgment, a logically probable outcome. Many also seek to hold others partly accountable for the infection or its consequences. Spirituality and morality help to address issues of responsibility and fate, and offer hope.

SIX

Missions: *Work and Volunteerism*

AS A RESULT of this illness, work takes on new forms and meanings. For many patients, volunteering for HIV-related organizations replaces previous employment and provides purpose, identity, and a means of contributing to others after one's own death. Infected individuals, based on their backgrounds and experiences, choose different types and functions of work and volunteerism.

The Dinosaur

Because jobs often serve as a locus of both professional and social lives, the loss of employment can cause profound distress. The prospect of disability benefits, precluding other employment, creates ambivalence. As Roy Gifford said, "I have mixed emotions about stopping work now in my forties. I have that old Puritan outlook that says, 'Work until you drop.' I try to do things on my own and wait for the day when I finally become ill and can't push myself any further—dropping dead in the harness. That's what my father and grandfather did. To retire early is giving up, and I've already given up enough things to HIV. I don't want people to notice that I'm not up to my old standard. I'd lose face. I've never applied for entitlements and don't intend to.

"The one time I didn't go along with my doctors was when I didn't retire last year, which they wanted me to do. I was trying to retain some dignity. I'll be damned if I'm going to be defeated. In my family, value is measured by the amount of work you do. Even old people do something, if only shelling beans. I have certain standards that I will not fall below, and retiring early is lowering my standards.

"I had no great designs to travel to the moon, but I wanted at least to outlive my granddads and uncles because it isn't right for the older generation to bury the younger. You're supposed to hit ninety. That's the ultimate goal."

Roy sees his own failure in cultural, not just personal, terms. His death carries added weight because of what else he feels will die with him. "I'm the last of the line, and I'm sad the tradition won't go on. The culture's dying out. Recently, when I referred to things that had been commonly spoken of at my grandmother's, my cousin had no idea what I was talking about." More will die than just himself. "I'm a survivor, the last of an old Dutch, Hudson Valley family that goes back ten generations. When I last saw my aunt, before she died of stroke, she came out of a coma, looked at me, pointed to herself, then to me, and said, 'Last Mohican Dinosaur.' Then she lay back down and became comatose again.

"Retirement has destroyed my plans. The relative importance of things had to change. All my life I thought, 'Why spend money when I might need it for something tomorrow?' In retrospect I should have done what I wanted, because tomorrow came anyway.

"I feel cheated. Nothing I do is ever enough. When I go into a pharmacy and buy two thousand dollars' worth of drugs, I look at them and think they'll only last one month. No matter how many pills I take, I'm not going to get rid of this disease. I just threw out my bank books. I looked at the accounts and thought, with all this money I could have had one hell of a good time, instead of being frugal and saving away for 'that wonderful day.' " He must come to terms with wide-ranging implications of the disease.

"When I told a friend recently that I might retire, he didn't handle it well. He felt I was giving in. He can't quite accept that I might get ill. He hasn't been 'out' that long or known people who have been ill. When I talk about it, he gets very quiet. The tone of his voice changes. His eyes get misty. He swallows hard and excuses himself from the room.

"My sense of time has also changed. I went from being very scheduled and rigid to being very unscheduled and unstructured, especially now that I'm not working. I don't have to be in an office by a certain time. I do my morning injections at 6:30 a.m., and my next obligation is to take a pill at eleven. Everything in between is filler. I clean the apartment, walk the dogs, care for the plants, go for a walk."

Partly as a result, Roy and others come to volunteer. "When I decided to retire, I thought that if I became depressed, I'd be sunk. So I started thinking about constructive things. I didn't want to spend all my life on AIDS-related activities, so I had to think what to balance them out with. What were my interests? What could I get involved with? I came up with doing volunteer work at the Botanical Garden and being a baby coddler. My lover was volunteering at the hospital, holding infected babies after they're born, before they're placed in foster homes. We feed them, rock them, and talk to them. I've also become involved with AIDS groups. Every Monday night I help with a supper for HIV-positive people in a Quaker church near me. I've become involved at a local more than a GMHC level." Volunteerism in fact constitutes Roy's main form of participation in HIV-land. His family had for generations remained in the same place, just outside New York City, tied to the land. Now he too is engaged with his neighborhood, not across the city.

His volunteerism is informal as well as formal. "I help others with AIDS. We keep track of each other. I call up and rattle them a little: 'Did you remember your appointment? Why not? Don't forget it tomorrow.' I do it because there is a need, a purpose. And without that, why go on?"

The Consultant

Others, unable to work full-time because of HIV, work or consult part-time, often through affiliations with their previous jobs. Such efforts become central components of their adaptation to the illness. Maurice Bradford, the former hospital administrator, told me, "I stopped work two months ago because symptoms increased. I was feeling weak. But I had also seen people stop working and have a good time before they died. Not fun, but they took advantage of the time they had. I didn't want to go from my desk, shuffling a lot of meaningless papers, to a hospital bed to a casket. I thought there could be something in between. So I stopped work, ending my career, cashing in on the dream I had of moving on to some job where I could make an impact in an organization. But it's been hard. I still drop by the office. It's painful to see that after two months things are happening that would not have occurred if I had been there. People are doing things in ways that are not particularly productive or useful. Whenever a department lacks a director or acting head, its turf gets attacked.

"I also consult now. My replacement calls and asks me things. I give lots of advice. I've provided some assistance informally, but he also arranges for small consulting fees for me. My disability program provides only 50 percent of my former income. It might have been easier just to sever my ties with my office and walk away. I try to think, 'Who gives a shit how a time sheet is filled out? Why should I worry about it?'

"But work has always been extremely important to me. I was never a person who watched the clock and worked only nine to five. I always put in a lot more time—uncompensated—than I had to. It was an important part of defining my life. Work was an escape from other things. If I was in a stressful relationship, it was easier to stay at work a little longer and put in a little more time. Or if I was not involved in a relationship, I'd spend time working into the evenings rather than sit home watching television. I liked the praise that came from doing a good job. When I slip into moments of existential angst, work helps define and shape who I am and reinforces my identity and sense of myself. In a world where I occasionally wonder what it's all about, it was nice to say, partly, that it was about drafting policies, managing people, and administering programs. That provided some meaning. I think of the jerks I've met who have no meaning in their lives. I look back at some of the people who gave me a hard time in high school, and I think, they're department store clerks while I've accomplished something meaningful and substantial. In a short period of time I achieved a relatively high administrative position and had the potential for more." Yet his statement that he "had" the potential also suggests the sense of loss he still feels, and the difficulty he has had giving it up.

"The importance of work to me stems largely from my experiences growing up gay," Maurice explained. "I had one good friend who was—to the extent that you can talk about it in ninth grade—a lover. He was on the football team, so nobody gave me a hard time. Then in the middle of my junior year, he dropped me without explanation and told everybody I was sucking his cock. Nobody suspected him of being interested. It was funny but extremely painful, and a terrible challenge. It was a tremendous character-building experience. In the early sixties an upstate New York Catholic high school wasn't really open to diverse lifestyles. I was harassed and taunted by people whom I thought were close friends. I'd ask a girl out for a date and she would back off, or break the date after people asked her, 'Why are you going out with that queer?' I learned to be alone, rely on myself, not worry that I didn't have friends, and function in a setting where I was isolated. I was degraded, ostracized, called names. It was not easy to go on. I couldn't talk to my parents or any adult.

"But I could impress teachers. They were my sanctuary. So at fifteen, rejected by my peers, I functioned and did exceptionally well. I turned my energy into doing a better job in school, and learned to be more alone with myself. That experience has helped me deal with all the things that came later. When I'm really challenged, I flash back to the horror of being rejected at fifteen and having no one to talk to. Ten years ago, when I was still upstate, I lost a job simply because I was gay. It made me stronger. No matter how emotionally painful something has been since, I have gotten through it. Before, I was weak.

"So I built a certain self-confidence that has helped in approaching HIV, caring for my lover. I didn't collapse in hysteria as some would have. On the job, too, I've been very strong. After years of supervising dozens of people, I still rate myself as more capable of coping with stress and pressure than most people I've worked with. I've developed an ability to define and analyze a problem and not exaggerate or distort it by my own fears. I'm pretty resourceful with solutions to management, work, and relationship problems—good at seeing options.

"So stopping work was a big deal for me. I also volunteer now at an AIDS organization that provides housing for homeless people with AIDS. I have two significant assignments. First, I answer the switchboard for one shift in the middle of the day. It's tangible and practical, a tough job with a dozen lines. When I do it I feel good because someone hasn't had to be paid to waste their time sitting at the switchboard. I'm also acting as a consultant, assessing their personnel management system or lack thereof. I have experience analyzing these situations. So it's exciting for me. I have found the meaning I used to get from my job. I spend fifteen hours a week with this organization.

"I also spend another five hours a week doing research studies, mostly at the hospital where I used to work. So I've put together a support structure and gotten the ability to call people, even from the organization where I volunteer. I've participated in studies from the beginning, mostly to make a contribution. But there's also a personal benefit—having access to researchers and getting information and more opinions. I'm in four different AIDS studies. It makes me feel better, dealing with these issues and with people who are trying to make sense of this whole thing and put it together to come up with some answers. As part of one research study, I inject into my body a substance the effects of which nobody yet knows. I also have huge tiers of P24 antibody. It's not clear if that's good or not, but it has seemed good enough to justify taking five hundred cc's of my plasma and passing it around every month through a research study. It seems to make people better." He thus volunteers literally both sweat and blood.

"Even after I die, my insurance will be used to make an impact, not just reward my family. I've designated significant contributions in my will to charitable AIDS organizations because I want to make a mark.

"I'm also still organizing my life, which is going to take forever. Applying for disability programs is a career in itself. Even I had no concept of what's entailed. Doctors, employers, and I all fill out forms.

"Some people say being HIV positive has just opened up their lives. I don't buy that. I understand how it changes one, but I'd rather do away with all of that and have the virus out of my system. HIV is the worst thing that could have happened to me at this point in my life." Those who say HIV provides benefits generally have less to lose, and have invested less in their futures.

Still, partly by having an outlet through volunteerism, Maurice avoids utter despair. "When I look back, I don't have many regrets. My life has been very full. I've learned a lot, traveled, experienced challenges, done some interesting work, and had very good friends and three significant love relationships. And I'm still trying to make a contribution."

Gay men, usually without children, often seek to leave something behind through their occupation. While Maurice established a career in health care, many gay men pursue the creative arts—film, theater, dance, writing, sculpture, or painting—which provide a bridge toward the future as well as an expression of feelings of difference and dissonance with the culture at large. Yet not everyone possesses talent in these areas or has time for them. As Jason Gillian, the Roman Catholic gay man, said, "I'm not a particularly creative person, though I try to be creative in how I live"—surviving in New York City, single, gay, and HIV-infected. Coming out, both as gay and as HIV positive, demands recreating the self.

The Agent: Becoming a Volunteer

HIV has also given a career and direction to some who lacked these before. Kerry Musgrove, who now holds a paid job at an AIDS organization, said, "After the epidemic began, following years of working for a theatrical agent, I went back to school to get a social work degree and began working for an AIDS agency. I was thirty-eight.

"What helps me now is having been an AIDS volunteer for so many years. When I started in '83, I had no idea I would ever have AIDS. It's still a surprise to me.

"I was not part of the gay community and didn't have a lot of gay friends, though working in the theater I knew a lot of gay people. But I remember thinking that to help out with the disease would be good—a way of broadening my life and helping other people, which I had not done before. But what really pushed me into it was that my ex-lover moved out. I was a basket case, totally devastated, a mess. I couldn't stop crying. I thought, 'If I do something to get me outside of myself, maybe it will help me, and perhaps somebody else too.' If it was just to benefit myself it wouldn't have lasted very long.

"It saved me. I had been working in this horrible theater job that paid $150 a week. I didn't know what I was going to do with my life.

"That's why I'm very grateful, not that AIDS is there, but that it has worked out the way it has. It led me into new career and personal areas, and I'm sure my life would not be as together now if I hadn't had these experiences. That's another reason why I continue to feel I have things to give back and why I like doing them.

"One thing I've had to figure out is where to put my anger. I went to ACT-UP meetings but couldn't stand being in a room of five hundred people screaming and bitching. It's too much random anger. Some of ACT-UP is sensational: they're brilliant at manipulating the media, and I'm thrilled they're there. The more political activism the better. But some is half-cocked; they don't know what they're doing. I can't get too involved because I get too frustrated. So I do my own thing. I try to channel my anger into work rather than public displays. That doesn't mean I don't do political things. But for me, the micro level is easier to deal with than the macro. It's easier for me to focus on individual people or small groups that need help—I feel I'm moving something along. I don't do well with committees or large groups or crowds. It helps me to break it down into small, workable units.

"People are amazed and ask how I could have had AIDS for two and a half years and still work with other PWAs around me all the time. I'm not entirely sure how I do it. And I do sometimes want to be more taken care of myself. But the work doesn't hurt me because I find it rewarding, and I think I do it well. I feel vulnerable anyway, so nothing else really makes it worse. I don't overidentify with other people's illnesses, even though I certainly am sympathetic. In some ways I am hurt by it. When a close colleague died—and I knew he was going to—I was still devastated. I don't think he'll ever be replaced in my life. But I'm still here. And I've finally accepted that this is who I am—a person who does these things."

One reason volunteerism helps Kerry is that he lacks other means of feeling part of something larger than himself. "I'm not at all religious. I was brought up Catholic, but if anything I'm agnostic. I stopped believing when I was seventeen."

He looks to modern physics to support his spiritual beliefs. "I think that when you're dead you're dead. But I also believe in physics, that energy doesn't die and that something of who we are will continue in some way, though we don't know what it is. It could be anything. I don't believe in a religious concept of God as a patriarchal figure sitting up there saying rock music is bad for you. But I also don't necessarily think it's total oblivion forever—a black hole—because there aren't any black holes in the universe."

The Tiniest Things Alive

Even for inner-city residents who have spent much of their lives in poverty, volunteering for HIV organizations serves important functions. HIV volunteerism is high among all socioeconomic groups and occurs for different reasons.

Several women who cannot connect with their own children, or have no children of their own, volunteer to help AIDS orphans. Olana Ramirez, who feared disintegration, said, "I handled jail and my husband's death, but I could not have handled my daughter being positive. The guilt alone. Just waiting for the results after she was born, I prayed, 'Oh God, please don't.' I vowed I would kill myself if she was positive. As it was, she was not going to have a daddy or mommy. That thought alone messed me up. Her father had been killed. God forbid I get sick and die, I'm afraid she'd have hardly any memories of me. I wouldn't see her grow up. I'd have left her and she wouldn't have a daddy, a brother, or a mother. That hurt. How can I let her be so little and hurt so much? Six years old and already seeing so much ugliness. How can I have infected her and given her more pain?

"Yet, thank God, she got tested and came out negative.

"She motivates me now when I feel weak. I think, 'God, please give me more time.' I want to give her something good to hold on to. She's a very strong motivation for me to keep clean.

"My mother left me when I was a little girl, and I lived with my grandparents until I was six. They raised me and gave me a lot of love. But I always wanted a daddy and a mommy. In school other kids called me a bastard. On Mother's Day I used to see all the other mothers, and I would bring my flower to my grandmother, but I would always cry. When I got to this country my biggest dream was that I was going to meet my mother and father and sister. But when I met my mother, it was like looking at a stranger. My sister was white with red hair, and I asked, 'Where's my father?' The man here turned out to be my stepfather, and nobody wanted to tell me who my real father was. The man here told me, 'I gave you a last name, but I didn't make you.' That hit me hard. I used to look out of my window at night and talk to the moon and the stars.

"When I got tested I thought, 'Shit. I should just start using drugs and end it.' But then I thought, 'God, I've got my kids.' They are everything to me and stop me from doing a lot of things.

"Now I do volunteer work on a ward where all the children are HIV. I do it first because I'm a recovering addict. Most of the mothers were addicts. A lot leave their babies and go out and pick up again, and their babies are born with the virus! I see little babies with IVs in their arms, and it hurts. I used needles and earned mine. I put myself in that position and can't blame anybody. If I hadn't shot dope, I wouldn't have AIDS. But what did little kids do? What did people that got infected from blood transfusions do? What did women whose husbands fooled around and gave it to them do? That's scary. Nobody can say it can't happen to them. I volunteer because I want to feel all this. And feel better about myself. I play with the kids and make them laugh. I always see one or two of the kids who come to me and we talk and play with the turtles. For some reason I'm good with kids. I can make them smile and give them a little warmth. They need it. They're the tiniest things alive and they're just left there. They need that warmth, not just bottle feeding. They need people to care for them. And I want to do that.

"The staff at my residence are worried about the stress level. They ask me about when the baby dies. 'What are you going to do? How are you going to deal with that? That'll break you.' My answer was that I would hurt because I'm a human being, but I'm going to have to learn how to separate. If I made that baby laugh, or happy, and made a difference in his life, I'm okay. I would be worse if I never brought a smile to that face. If I cry, I'll cry. I'm not gonna hold back. But I want to do this work. Hopefully I'll be able to. I believe that God doesn't give you something you can't handle.

"I also speak with the mothers because I feel their pain. I admire mothers that stay with their kids, and I feel badly for the mothers that knew they were positive before they got pregnant. How could they have taken a chance like that with another life? But the ones I feel the worst for are the ones that didn't know beforehand. They may have never used drugs. It may have been their husband's fault." Volunteer work thus serves several functions for Olana, in part enabling her to expiate her own guilt toward her children.

Many who volunteer and "give back" to the HIV community in fact receive disability, obviating other employment and allowing them free time. Government benefits thus indirectly augment the services provided to others with HIV. Yet many who are still working also volunteer.

Religious activism often serves as a model for HIV-related volunteer work. "I have a mission to teach others about HIV," Gregory Colson, who found religion while in prison, said. "Now I spread the word, not the virus. In a way I'm glad I have it. Everybody has a mission or path or reason for which they came into this world. One of my reasons is not just to suffer but to be an example and give knowledge to other people. That is why I stay alive. It gives me a purpose. I lecture to groups and petition the government to reform the treatment of HIV-positive prisoners. The Lord will guide me as long as I do his work." Gregory's volunteerism allows for moral reconciliation, making up for past misdeeds. Yet his striving comes at a price. "It's insurance," he says, "but when will I know if I have done enough?"

Volunteerism is not for everyone. As Roy Gifford commented, "I don't think I could be a buddy in one of these systems where people just volunteer to help people they don't know. Somebody I loved, like one of my friends, I would, because I loved them. But that would be it." Instead he focuses on other avenues and his pets—who are healthy and alive.

These forms of work follow from experiences before and since infection. The end of a career can mean the dissolution of dreams, priorities, and links to the future. But work can also soften the impact of losses from the disease. Volunteerism provides a variety of benefits—a way of acting constructively against the virus, establishing new connections to the future, and redeeming perceived misdeeds. Despite the difficulties of living with HIV, many patients help others, responding altruistically in times of trouble and contributing to something beyond themselves. Work becomes a mission.

SEVEN

Recovering Parents: *Connections with Families*

TO COUNTER the destruction and stigma of HIV, many infected individuals seek to reconnect with kin. This goal allows men and women to "live on" after death through future generations. Yet, given past difficulties, the reestablishment of such bonds can pose enormous obstacles and create new strains.

A Pact with God

Like Olana Ramirez, the major issues Gerry Galvez has faced over time involve her children. Gerry, whom the orderly had eventually stopped visiting in the hospital, explained, "I found out I was pregnant while in prison. I came home from Rikers Island seven months pregnant and had nowhere to live. I have a family and don't have a family. They exist. I have a mother and father and three sisters. But they don't want anything to do with me. When I was on drugs I was the lowest thing and wasn't allowed in their house. They wouldn't talk to me. I was homeless with no source of income and had my two-year-old son with me.

"I used to pickpocket and shoplift. That's what I had gotten arrested for. But I decided I had had enough of that. So I was sleeping in hallways and wherever the night would catch me. I would sit, taking handouts. But I had made up my mind not to do anything that would make me go back to jail or lose my baby. So I slept on rooftops. It was bitter, bitter cold, and I'd cover my two-year-old son with newspapers to keep him warm. A homosexual who lived in the building told me about a little room with a sink and a lock. He said, 'Wait until late at night. We could open the lock and go in. You can stay there.'

"After I gave birth to my daughter, I started smoking crack and getting really depressed. I would just sit there and look at my newborn baby and think about her dying. That's when I suddenly saw she wasn't breathing and I ran to the hospital. They kept her in the hospital and gave her antibiotics. But she wouldn't respond.

"That's also when I got tested. At the time I thought only homosexuals got HIV. That's as far as I knew. But I signed the papers, and they drew blood from my baby and told me it would take three to four weeks to get the results. When the results came back, I had no address and the doctor couldn't get in touch with me. One morning my mother came with a letter from the doctor telling me to call the hospital. I called and the doctor said, 'Come to my office first thing tomorrow morning. It's very important.' So I kind of got the idea.

"The doctor told me to sit down, that both my test and my baby's were positive. But my baby might be positive just because she had my antibodies, so there was a possibility she would convert to negative. I was hurt, but for my baby, not for me. I felt like it should be me that dies. I prayed to God: take me but give my little baby a chance to live. At least I was thirty-four, I had had some years."

Her feelings arise partly from her past. "I had lost my first daughter to the city. I was fifteen years old at the time and had no say. She was born preemie and was in an incubator. All I did was look at her through the window. I never even got to feed or touch her. They told me I would be able to take her home, and I held on to that. I would watch the nurses taking care of my baby through the window. One morning they called my mother and said she could take my baby home. That was the biggest thing in the world for me. I had just turned fifteen. I had bought a crib and all this stuff and set it up in the front room of my mother's house. I was pickpocketing at the time, and paid my mother to stay there.

"But when I got to the hospital, some men looking like detectives were there, and the social worker told me she wanted to speak with me. She said they couldn't let me have my baby, that I had to go with them to take the baby to the Foundling Hospital. I begged the social worker to call my mother, because the only way they wouldn't take the baby away was if my mother took it. But my mother said she had already raised her children and wasn't going to raise mine. So they took my baby away, and I went and had an overdose to try to kill myself.

"Someone I used to get high with found me. He had seen me going up on this skylight. So he saved my life. I was out of it for about two days. When I came to, I looked in the mirror and was blue.

"So now, when I was waiting for my baby's HIV test result, I made a pact with God—please, if you let my baby become HIV negative and normal, I'll do whatever has to be done to pass the word on and see that people save themselves.

"Eventually my baby converted to HIV negative. It was a miracle. I realized then, though, that I had to stop IV drugs.

"But a few months later I went back to living with my common-law husband, and eventually he started giving me a hard time. All he was doing was living with me. So I said, 'Listen, it just can't work like this. We either work on bettering our relationship or you have to leave.' But he refused. Sex was the only kind of communicating he wanted. I would tell him, 'Look, you can't continue to have sex unless you wear a condom.' He would say, 'No, there's nothing wrong with you. Those doctors are full of shit. You're just faking. I'm not going nowhere.'

"So it got to the point where we weren't having sex. He got frustrated. 1990 had been a good year for us. I didn't push for safer sex, so everything was all right. But then one morning he got paid and I waited for him to give me some money. He got up, took a shower, and dressed. I asked, 'Where are you going?' He said, 'I found me somebody else. When you start doing the right thing, I'll give you some money.' I said, 'Man, you must be crazy! These kids gotta eat.' We started struggling. Finally I said, 'All right, I'm gonna go to the precinct, and you either get out or do what you're supposed to, or go to jail.' He was walking out the door. I said, 'And the next bitch that calls here, I'm gonna tell her that you have AIDS.' Then I closed the door behind him. That really got to him 'cause he stood there and said, 'Open the door, I have to get my bag.' I said, 'If you think that you're gonna come in here and put your hands on me and get away with it, I've got news for you.' He said, 'I'm not gonna do nothing to you, just open the door.' He was talking real nice. So I went and got a knife and stepped back into my son's room and opened the door. He walked in, and when I closed the door he grabbed me and started banging me against the wall and threw me down on the floor and started kicking my face. So I stabbed him. I took the whole knife and stuck it in his leg. He dragged himself a little bit and then fell and lost a lot of blood. The police came and put us both in jail for assault.

"Now I go to different conferences and talk about myself, and stand up for women—Latin women and women that are positive. I talk about what we're going through and how it's harder for women. I meet people now. I'm an activist. I had no self-esteem before, but now I feel good about myself. I'm proud of myself.

"A couple of women who got beaten up called me, crying, and I counseled them and helped them get into battered women's shelters. I ask them, 'What's most important? You are!'

"I'm glad I stopped drugs and got my life together and am there to take care of my kids." Given the enormous chaos and devastation she had earlier faced, she now seeks connection to her children and others.

No More Children

For those without children, HIV poses a different set of issues. For Jenny Singer, the nurse, "the worst part of HIV is not being able to have a child now. I always wanted to have children and raise a family, but I waited a long time—until I had straightened my life out. I'd been pregnant and had two abortions. Now that I have the virus, I can't get pregnant again. I know there's a chance I could have a seronegative child, but it would break my heart if I gave birth and then had to watch the child be sick for years and die from AIDS. I couldn't inflict that kind of pain on another human being. Instead I just bought a cute little baby dog. It's nice to see her growing and changing every day. No matter what I do or say, she always loves me. She depends on me daily and gives me hugs and kisses. I sing little poems to her, putting her name into the song. She loves it and goes nuts.

"My relationship with my family has also gotten stronger. I've been able to patch up a lot of relationships and bad feelings."

Audrey Baker, a forty-eight-year-old African-American woman, has older children. Still, "HIV means no future since I can't have another child now," she reported. She wants another child, in part out of guilt over not being available for her children because of her drug use.

"I got pregnant when I was eighteen," she explained, "and didn't know where babies came from. I thought they cut you and took the baby out. My mother never talked about things like that.

"This weekend I stayed with my niece, and my sister called every few hours, worried about her grandchild. The baby was calling my sister 'grandma.' I said, 'That would be nice to have a grandchild.' I'd love to see what my kids' kids would look like. That extending of myself, that extension. I would like to experience that kind of love for my daughter's baby. I can't have any more little babies. My kids are grown. But I love little babies. I wish sometimes I was able to have one more baby or somebody would give me a baby. I have a fantasy that someone will leave a baby for me in a paper bag. I know that's wrong to say, but that's how I feel. I would do things differently, stop a lot of things. I wouldn't drink and would get off methadone and do everything right—like before I started drugs."

HIV prompts men as well as women to seek connection through children. Reynaldo Fernandez, who felt his "seed" was "poison," elaborated. "The virus has this much over me: that it's not allowing me to have a kid in a normal way, or have sex freely without having to think whether I am going to expose the woman to the virus. Just knowing that it's not the normal procedure to get a woman pregnant, I feel less than a normal man. That's not to say I am less than a man, but it plays a big psychological part. It has to do with machismo. From my culture I inherited an attitude that a man's got to be a certain way or he isn't really a man. I know I'm a man. But the virus keeps me from being able to perform like any other normal man, which makes me feel bad. I'm coming to terms with it—that I'm not less, that it's just the virus. But I get very angry. All through my life I've always had to settle for seconds. I was never able to do what I really wanted. Maybe I didn't deserve to. I did everything the opposite of what my parents told me. If my father said, 'Don't hang out with this one,' I'd hang out with that one anyway."

Many gay men also wish they had had children. Raoul Rodriquez said, "I could have done a lot of things without HIV, maybe had a kid. I always had the idea of having a kid. I even made a woman pregnant once, but she aborted. Sometimes I think I didn't give that kid a chance to live. I'm dying, and what did I do? I want to have done something, built a relationship or had a child. I work and do things and make a decent salary. But I would like to be able to do something for a son or daughter. HIV stops me. All my life I wanted to have something that could give some sense to my life. I want to have a child because I feel lonely. If I had someone to work for, all my problems would be reduced. What am I working for? Simply to buy food in a nice restaurant and see movies? A kid would give me something, someone to work for. I don't really have anybody. Adopting a child is not the same thing, though I know other gays who do it."

Gay men without children often seek to establish relationships with nieces and nephews. For example, one gay man and his lover, both with AIDS, built a doll house for an infant niece, for her to remember them by when she got older. The two men spent much of their remaining time over many months before they died carefully constructing it, furnishing it with miniature curtains, chairs, and tables they built themselves. They cut up and sewed in bits of their own clothes and furniture to be used in the house after they were gone.

The Grown Woman That's My Daughter

To reconnect with families and children after times of absence or neglect, significant barriers must often be overcome. Elsa Diaz, a thirty-eight-year-old Latina woman, has short light brown hair and a round face. "I haven't had a relationship with any of my children," she explained. "At twenty-three I had four children and picked up heroin. When it got real bad with arrests, I couldn't function and gave the children to my mother. So I've had sporadic relations with them. I'd come and see them or write them from jail. But there was really no relationship there. I would like to build a new one now, before it's over. But because they were raised by my mother, it's difficult. The oldest one lived with me for a time, but it was during my drug addiction and the whole thing. Being off drugs now, I'm like a kid. My daughter moved in with me seven months ago, and I don't know what to say to her. I'm in a house with a grown woman that's my daughter, but I don't know her. It's been insane. Someone even told her she shouldn't be with me because I could influence her recovery.

"I still don't know how to express what I feel to her. It gets very emotional, and I just break down and cry. I've never raised no children. I give little opinions, but my kids are looking for me to do something that I don't know anything about. Last night I was stressed out because she's into doing her hair and had bought fake hair and braided it on her head, and pieces of hair were all over the house. I'm used to being by myself and having everything just so, and I had to tell her I was very tired and can't sleep if my house is junky.

"She had been moving from place to place, not eating properly and starting to drink again. I told her, 'You can come here and do what you supposed to do. You got ninety days to show me that you gonna do something.' I felt I owed her that, to take her off the street.

"I feel like I'm a mother with all of them. But I'm just not capable yet of expressing my love and concern because I've lived such a wild life myself. I'm not used to telling somebody what to do. All my life I just had me. When I was dealing with drugs, everything was okay. I'd get me a drug and I was happy. So I understand very well what they're going through. Sometimes I hesitate to say to them, 'Don't do that because of the repercussions,' because they answer back, 'Well *you* did it.' 'And you see what happened to me.' Throughout my life people told me, 'You shouldn't do this and that.' But my mind told me, 'It ain't gonna happen to me like it happened to you.' Only it happened worse. So a lot of times I hesitate to tell them, 'You shouldn't do that.' It's a pain within myself: will they like me? But I've decided, it ain't about them liking me but about telling them the truth." Elsa and other parents who have stopped drugs and become more available to their children discover they have problems because they have so little experience raising children.

"My daughter sits in classrooms and discusses the virus and other kids tell her, 'People with the virus should be put on an island somewhere.' Even my mother told my children they shouldn't be around me, they could get sick. My mother is a psychiatric registered nurse who tends to AIDS patients and knows that's an out and out lie.

"I had lost my youngest son because in the hospital I had admitted I was an addict. They had threatened to take him, and then one day I got to the hospital and he was gone. I died. I felt dead. That weekend I shot drugs and drank, trying to erase the pain because it seemed like life wasn't worth living. I couldn't see my son, and they told me I was disabled. It seemed my entire life had been a waste. I laid there and prayed, let me die.

"A lot of times I've gone into court, which is very painful. It's been hinted to me that because I was a substance abuser and have AIDS, I don't need my son, and he's better off without me. The family court system discriminates against HIV-positive parents. The agency that governs his foster care is neglectful because a foster parent wants him. But my God, who are they and who made them? I have an overwhelming desire to be reunited with my son, and I must stay alive to do that. The fact that I can't see him is the most painful thing I can think of. I see other little children, and it's hard.

"The lawyers advise me that I shouldn't tell the court I'm HIV positive—because then I'll never get him—or say that I fear I might die before the judge decides. I can do for my son what was not done for me, and give him a chance. But they feel the separation is better for him, even though I know it's not. That alone is killing me." Her son is important to her, not just for a sense of life extending beyond her but for her dignity, given the shame she feels because of her past. She also wants to make things up to him, given her earlier absence.

Elsa confronts difficult issues surrounding the future custody of her children. "My brother calls every other day since he found out I'm HIV positive, and asks me if I want to join him on everything he does—picnics, movies, dances. 'How you doing? You're okay? You're not sick?' I say, 'I'm okay.' He would never call me before. When my phone got disconnected, he gave me the money for it. He talked to me about doing a will to leave my youngest daughter to him. I said, 'Wait a minute. I'm not dying.'" She resists arranging custody because it means she must come to terms with death.

To reestablish links with children is often one of the major tasks an infected parent faces. For Lorraina Ortiz, for example—whose son arranged a meeting between her mother and herself—relationships with family lie at the crux of her problems in dealing with HIV. Her daughter was raised by Lorraina's sister; now both want nothing to do with Lorraina. "Right now my only child I speak to is my youngest son. The last time I spoke to my daughter was Christmas. I write to her but she doesn't answer. She can't accept it. She feels I wasn't there when she needed me, and won't be there in the future. She can't talk about me in school. She would have to come out and say, 'My mother was an addict and has AIDS.' If you ask her about her mother, she says, 'My mother lives in New

York. I'm not in contact with her.' She wants to keep it that way, which hurts. Sometimes my feelings are mixed—hatred for myself and even for my kids, because they can't understand that whatever I went through happened. But I'm still their mother. I'm not saying they have to accept it, but they should still be there for me. Sometimes I hate my daughter because she can't accept that I'm sick and need her. It's wrong, but that's how I feel. I've spoken to her about it. She says it could happen to somebody else's mother but not to hers. She's getting married but doesn't want me to meet her fiancé's parents. She says, 'My mother is lost, gone.'

"She also pulls my youngest son away from me. He tells me, 'She wants me just to forget about you. You're going to die, so we might as well say you're dead already.' But she is making matters worse for me, because it hurts, and then because of all that stress I want to pick up drugs again. The only thing that holds me back is knowing that if I go out there and use drugs, I'll probably never come back. I'll develop AIDS. It will get to a point where I won't be able to deal with my addiction and will probably end up killing myself. I'd have nothing to live for.

"Luckily I have a gay brother who works in ACT-UP and GMHC and is very supportive. He is the only one I have in my family."

Many parents face resentment, not only from their children but from their own parents and siblings. Dede Alwin's mother, who had sent Dede to a Catholic boarding school, now has to raise Dede's son. Dede accepts the arrangement: "God forbid if something happens to me, he'd go in foster care and they'd find out his mother had the virus. Who knows how they'd treat him? I don't want that. So my mother takes care of him. I messed up with cocaine and drinking, and to have my mother take care of my son is a disappointment for her. She's getting older, and taking care of a six-year-old is not easy. She's retired and wants to relax and enjoy life. Instead she's thinking about this kid. She has to keep him and take care of his clothes and food. She doesn't want her grandchild to be put up for adoption. She'll love him the best she can. She's very religious. She just said, 'Well . . .', and closed up on it. I had a dream about a week ago that I was someplace in the mountains and the water was crisp and I had my son. I remember this brook, the water flowing. I could hear sounds around me from animals, birds chirping. I felt good, refreshed. The sun was shining. The past couple of weeks my son has been in camp.

"I want him to be happy when I am gone. I always think of the gleam in his eye when he's happy. I want him to be an engineer, dealing with computers. But as long as he turns out to be good and honest. He likes life—so far anyway. I want to prevent him from making a lot of mistakes I made."

Gloria Higgens, in the AIDS residence, looked for a moral explanation for her difficulties with her son. "My son is having a real hard time dealing with my having AIDS. He doesn't want to believe it. He's not ashamed of me. He tells all his friends, 'Yes, my mother has AIDS, but she looks good and gets around well.' He's not afraid to walk the street with me.

"For years he didn't know what was going on with me. Nobody knew where I was, because I wasn't in touch with my family until after I had been sick in the hospital. All the time he was in prison I never called or visited him, because I was running the street, drugging. The last time I saw his father, my son was seven years old.

"When situations with my son are difficult, I feel I'm getting back what I did to my mother. A lot of what I go through with him repeats what happened with her and me. It makes me think a lot about her. My mother was a real hell-fighter. Everybody loved her. She was strong—with all the shit she went through with us. I miss her. But she's looking down on me and sees that I'm trying. Before she passed, she said she wanted me to get my son out of the block where he was living, and get my life together. It's really important that I do that." Her son provides a chance for redemption.

Recovering Grandparents

Many HIV patients look to a future generation—to grandchildren—as an opportunity to start a clean slate. Eddie Lourdes, who felt God has given him a second chance, said, "Some people's goal will be reached twenty years from now. But I can't wait that long. So my little goal is at least to see my grandkids. My daughter will be twelve and my son eleven. If I see my grandkids I could die satisfied. At least I will have seen something mine. That would make me feel good, like I was there. I was fifteen years old when I had my daughter and my son. Now my son is a man. If I live long enough to see grandchildren, I'll know I'll have done my job. I can go and die in peace. I'd have finished raising them. I pray: "Let me see my grandkids, then take me. Give me my grandkids and I'll stay clean. The only thing I want to do is see them. I promise you, God, I'll do the right thing, stay out of trouble.' It's a deal with God." Eddie bargains to ease his moral conflict. Grandchildren would provide a sense of continuity, offering proof that his children succeeded by having children of their own. Although Eddie feels he was not a good parent, his children thus would be.

"The most difficult part of HIV is thinking about leaving my family and wondering how my kids will be when they get older," he adds. "My brother and I disappointed our mother. I did time in jail. I want to make it up to my kids now. It's not easy. I want to teach them now what I wanted to teach them three years ago. But now they already know it. I try to spend more time with them. I want to make up for lost time and future time. I lost ten years in jail. Afterward I didn't want my kids to see me on drugs, nodding off, so I spent more time by myself and with my friends. Being HIV positive, I don't have much hope of gaining more years.

"Pretty soon they're going to start going out to parties. I want to be there for them. My father wasn't there when I started to party. If he was, things could have been a lot different. I wouldn't have gone to drugs.

"My three brothers and I are all HIV positive. Each of us wants to go first. We don't want to see my mother watching the other two of us dying, one at a time.

"Seeing grandkids would be like seeing my kids born again, something of mine, my material. My son and my son's kids will carry my name. But I can't tell them that's my goal. I don't want grandkids as a favor to me. My daughter would probably go out and have a baby just so I can see a grandchild. So I keep it inside."

Beatrice Rosaro, a forty-five-year-old Latina and former drug user, has grandchildren but still faces problems. "I want to better myself, not be an addict with a grandchild. It wouldn't look nice, pushing a baby carriage, high. I want to be a recovering grandmother, take him to the park, the store, walk with my head up proud. I feel he knows who I am. I'm not a stranger to him. Having grandchildren makes me feel I'm needed, useful. I take them outside. But there was a time when my daughter wouldn't even let me see my grandson. She didn't want him around me because she knew I was smoking crack. My kids ain't stupid. My daughter lived in the same building, and I was in there getting high."

Many gay men felt estranged from their families even before HIV, but they have no easy possibility of children or grandchildren as a means of making amends for the past or achieving closure. For these men, the arts and volunteerism often provide possible connections to others and to the future.

Many gay men's parents even refuse to accept their son's homosexuality. Some families have "disowned" sons who came out. Roy Gifford said, "At Christmas I spoke to my mother—the Wicked Witch of the West—because of some family dealings. It was the first time I had spoken with her in five years. Her opening comment was, 'I'm surprised you're still alive. I thought you were dead.' I concluded the family business and hung up. My mother and I had been very close until I came out. She and I supported the household. My brother lived at home and contributed nothing.

"I had collected $500,000 worth of antiques, but when I had an auctioneer come who knew the caliber of the stuff, the boxes were empty. When I questioned my mother, she claimed the stuff never existed. Seventeen years of my life were flushed down the toilet. When my father died I was supposed to get the house and the property. My brother got the business, which he bankrupted. When my mother sold the house, she gave him all the assets. I ended up dealing with my family only through attorneys."

Yet gay men, when sick, often have no choice but to reconnect with their families of origin. Many, forced to return home because of illness or finances, face conflict and frustration. Ken Landers, the actor who has had to move back in with his parents, fights with them incessantly. "They watch every little movement I make. If I go out, they want to know where I'm going and when I'm coming back. As a result, I sometimes feel like slapping my mother." They put him in the sick role and see him as dying, but he does not view himself this way.

Families can provide bridges to the future, but not always easily. Such connections operate both physically through genes and symbolically through improvements in the lives of future generations. These efforts can counter long-standing vicious cycles of poverty and addiction. Yet families can also be distancing, unforgiving, and unwilling to aid infected members. Such barriers may prove insurmountable. Attempts to be closer to kin may frustrate or fail, exacerbating stress and prompting searches for other connections, or escape.

EIGHT

No Big Deal

INSTEAD OF ADAPTING in the ways we have seen, many men and women choose a different course: they attempt to soften the impact of HIV by minimizing the virus's effects. To make the diagnosis less devastating, they reframe the disease—for example, acknowledging one stage of their HIV-spectrum disorder but not another.

Only Positive

"I'm only HIV positive," Arthur Williams told me. An African-American gay man, he arrived in my office wearing red shorts, a black T-shirt, stylish boots, and a baseball cap, the brim tilted sideways off his head. He had worked as a striptease artist and a hustler. "If I were AIDS positive," he explained, "I'd be depressed and probably want to kill myself. But since I'm only HIV positive, I'm okay, and the virus doesn't bother me." Yet in fact he met the criteria for AIDS, having had Kaposi's sarcoma, a major opportunistic infection.

"I'm only twenty-one and have my whole life ahead of me. I've seen what AIDS has done to people, and I don't want to end up like that. It devastates people, and I wouldn't want to see me in that state. If I knew I was going to wither away, I would just get rid of myself. I want people to remember me the way I am, not the way I'd look before I die. I'm very proud of how my body looks. I like to wear T-shirts and tight things and show myself off. I work out every day. When I was younger I was fat. My father used to beat me up and then kicked me out of the house for being gay. I grew up thinking I was very ugly. I feel much better about myself now. I know this might sound superficial to some people, but the fact that guys in the street cruise me now makes me feel worthwhile.

"So I try not to look at the fact that I'm HIV positive. I try to look at myself as still a human being. I don't look in terms of HIV: am I HIV positive or am I just positive? Whatever it comes out to be, I'll have to learn to accept it because I guess it was bound to happen, or there's nothing I can do about it. If I started sitting down and telling myself, 'Oh God, I'm HIV positive,' I would be one hell of a depressed person. I watch the shows about HIV on TV, but I don't like half of them because they don't show the right side—the very positive side of HIV—only the depressing side.

"I'm definitely not sick now, so I definitely don't consider myself sick. I consider myself as somebody who's infected. I try to keep a positive outlook on everything. Maybe they'll come up with a cure soon." Arthur's minimization stems in part from his experiences growing up.

His future fears also contribute. "If I developed AIDS, there would be nobody to take care of me. I would be alone, bedridden, helpless, unable to have somebody wipe my ass for me or help me use a bedpan. I try to present myself well, and even if I were sick I'd want my hair combed." The loss of bodily integrity, leading to a state similar to that during infancy, would thus be doubly humiliating. For Arthur and many gay men, whose sexual orientation has shaped their adult lives, the body and its potential decay can take on special importance.

Other personal factors can be involved in this reframing. As Ken Landers, who had to move in with his parents, said, "One day I noticed these little discolorations on my leg. I didn't want to think they were KS [Kaposi's sarcoma]. My image of KS and the term 'lesion' were a lot worse then these. To me a lesion is something open and puffy, and these weren't. But I showed them to a doctor friend who said, 'You know this is KS, don't you?' And I said, 'Well, yeah, I guess I do.' But I didn't really. I was upset, afraid everything was suddenly going to start falling apart. But then my doctor said that a lot of experts are not relating KS to HIV as much as they once did, and that KS isn't a diagnosis of AIDS anymore. He doesn't even really consider me ARC because I haven't had anything besides the KS. I don't know if he's just saying that to make me feel better, or if it's medically correct, but I definitely feel better. Now I don't classify myself as ill but as fine with just this bug in me. I've had only occasional symptoms, not enough to say, 'I'm going to die.' My bloods have always been good. So I don't have AIDS. I'm only HIV positive with a few symptoms, and I don't dwell on it."

Ken grew up in suburban New Jersey and had moved to New York to try acting while supporting himself as a word processor. His theater career foundered, and HIV forced him to give it up and return home to his parents. He feels he has not accomplished much in his life and that AIDS will deprive him of any future chance.

His denial continues at every stage of the disease process. "I've had sweats at night, but I attribute them to the crypto, not the HIV." He also redefines medical signs and symptoms. "I thought my T-cells were 500, the normal level. I found out they were only 276, which really freaked me out." He defines 500 as "normal" whereas it is in fact diminished.

Ken avoids not only the medical but the social, sexual, and psychological implications of HIV. "Initially KS was a pretty depressing thought. But more for vanity than for medical reasons. I thought, oh shit. I can't go out and have sex or be in a relationship now. People will look at me and say, 'Get away.' "

But he has trouble hiding his visible lesions. "When I went for a haircut I felt very sensitive about one spot on the back of my ear. A couple of times the haircutter said, 'Wow, what the hell is that on your ear?' And I said, 'I don't know. What is it?' He said, 'Man, it looks funny.' My friends said, 'Well, it's not *that* noticeable.' One on my eye was a lot larger, and I felt everybody saw it." Unmistakable lesions, revealing to others his diagnosis, make his minimization of the illness more difficult.

In the film *Philadelphia* the visibility of KS lesions marks both turning points in the plot: first when a law partner observes a purple spot on Tom Hanks's forehead, and second when Hanks pulls off his shirt in the courtroom, revealing splotches that signal him as truly diseased—winning him his court case but marking him as fated to die. Skin lesions become stigmata with profound social and psychological implications.

Ken's earlier experiences with illness fuel his current denial. In his early twenties he had Hodgkin's lymphoma, successfully treated. "Everyone around me was flipping out at the time. But there I was in the hospital getting radiation every day, and it wasn't a big deal to me. I wasn't interested in finding out more about it, so I didn't. I didn't really think I was going to die. They were just going to radiate me, and I'd be fine. So learning that I'm HIV positive hasn't been a big deal to me either. I accept it, having already gone through one sort of cancer. I figure if I get sick, they'll fix me again. If they can do anything, they will. If they can't, fine. Why go crazy over something you can't fix? I'm a very mellow, calm, low-key person, the type that holds stuff in rather than explodes. I just coast along and whatever happens, happens.

Man has found so many cures for awful diseases—eventually they'll find a vaccine or something that will either arrest the disease or just vanish it. Man will bring to bear on this enemy his basic ingenuity and powers of discovery. So unless I really become ill, I don't know if HIV will ever become a big part of my life. I don't think anything ever really does. My parents are totally the opposite and are very rigid. If it's six o'clock, they have to have dinner. I can almost tell the time by them."

New, improved treatments now are emerging, using protease inhibitors, yet individuals minimized their illness even before these new therapies were developed. Such minimization is important as a psychological defense.

Ken also avoids contemplating the virus by staying occupied. "I work at home as a freelance word processor, and when there's a low period I have much more time just to think. So I try to stay busy and not think about it, not get depressed."

He shies away from reminders that the illness can worsen. He dropped out of a support group "because some members were sicker and forced me to think about HIV every week. I also don't read many press reports about AIDS. They make me think more about HIV. Knowledge changes so much anyway. Sometimes I don't read *Science Times* because the following week the news will all be different anyway. For example, when Interferon first came out it was going to save everybody, but the following week further research showed it wasn't as wonderful as first thought. So I don't hang on every word in print. I notice articles but don't read them fanatically. TV shows on HIV are valuable for the rest of the population, but I don't like watching somebody in a hospital ward dying of AIDS."

Illness becomes ordinary in Ken's mind. "I've always had medical problems: mononucleosis in high school, then Hodgkin's, hepatitis a few years later, another strain of hepatitis after that, and now this. For me it's normal to have medical stuff, so I don't let it upset me. Besides, everybody goes through something."

He also normalizes the possibility of death in the near future. "I could walk out on the street and get hit by a Mack truck. So you never know. It doesn't have to be from HIV."

The newness of the disease and changes in its diagnostic criteria also promote confusion. "What are AIDS and ARC anyway?" he asks. "They're only words"—as if they correspond only to other words rather than to medical conditions.

Similarly he disparages alternative perspectives. "I'm not avoiding HIV in a bad way—at least I don't think I am. I'm just not thinking about it in order not to dwell on it and build it up even bigger than it really is. I have friends doing just the opposite. They're totally hypochondriacal about everything, and depressing to talk to. One friend of mine is an angry AIDS queen. It's hard to say *anything* to him."

Yet Ken's minimization causes problems. While he sees himself as "living with HIV," his family sees him as sick and dying. Forced to reside with them, he feels their concern is "overkill. They're constantly doting, watching me." Conflict is frequent.

He also practices sex that is less safe than that of many who are more disturbed by the disease. He engages in "fairly safe sex" that some would consider unsafe.

Other individuals employ additional strategies of minimization. Rodney Jones, a thirty-six-year-old African-American former injecting drug user, initially looked for reasons to believe he was in fact uninfected. "I was in prison, and they took blood tests. I was really under the impression that if they didn't segregate me or didn't tell me anything, I must be healthy." Even after learning of his infection, his lack of symptoms facilitated his minimization. "I'd seen people deteriorating in the last stages of ARC and full-blown AIDS, and I thought *that* was HIV. So I saw myself as healthy and said the results aren't right. I can't be HIV because I'm in good health." Wilma Smith also thought at first that a mistake had been made. These attitudes reflect the fact that HIV, as an externally applied label, can radically conflict with one's inner experience of oneself. Wilma thus had to see the lab results "in black and white." As noted earlier, some people avoid being tested at all or never pick up the results.

Yvette Bing, who hadn't picked up her test results, experiences symptoms but attributes them to sources other than HIV. "Everybody we were hanging out with was dying, one after the other. I got really scared. But I didn't do anything about it. I started getting sick, with chills and sweats at night, and I thought it was the drugs. They cut drugs with terrible things. My night sweats could also be due to methadone or my hysterectomy. I had low energy from the AZT, and anemia"—though anemia can result from HIV. "Besides, I only have a mild case," she adds, reconceptualizing the illness, though her symptoms warrant a diagnosis of what used to be called ARC. "And I can't do anything about HIV anyway, so why bother dwelling on it?" Yet she had also continued to use drugs and share needles, spreading the virus to others. Her minimization has thus served her desires, removing her from any urgency or responsibility to stop her drug behavior. It has allowed her to continue to spread the virus.

Yvette also reframes the illness, feeling she is "just a carrier unless I don't take care of myself. On paper I'm an HIV diagnosis, but that's it," she said, separating her diagnosis on paper from her experience. She constructs the illness as not being potentially fatal; she sees herself as a conduit, not a target. "Sometimes I don't even believe I have HIV. I don't feel different. I don't have symptoms of it. Because I don't feel sick, I'm not sick. Sometimes I feel like taking the test again because it might have been a mistake. It's probably somebody else's blood and they put my name on it. Sometimes they make mistakes. There are a lot of ifs. But that doesn't put me in denial or I'd be out there doing crazy things because I wouldn't want to accept it. I just can't lose sleep over it. Deep down I know I have it. I think about it once in a while, especially at night when I'm trying to get to sleep. I think about the future. But not every day."

Yvette's minimization fuels her continued substance use. "I don't really see nothing wrong in drinking beer. I don't see how it could hurt my immune system. It's not drugs. But then I also know that alcohol can do more damage than drugs. It's just that I can't deal with pressure: I get high. The longest period I was off drugs were my last two pregnancies. I didn't want to addict my baby."

Confusion about the illness promotes minimization. Gary Stevens, an African-American injecting drug user, said, "As far as I know, HIV is a blood disease—just a blood disorder, something in my system." He wants to believe the virus won't progress or lead to AIDS.

The presence or absence of symptoms in others can also shape an individual's minimization. "HIV doesn't bother me that much," George Sullivan said, "until people I know get sick or die." Then HIV troubles him intensely, but eventually his concern wanes until the next such crisis occurs. This shared response to medical symptoms is a unique feature of an epidemic.

Others accept the fact they are infected but feel their future will be unaltered. Roger Babson, the gay man in the AIDS residence, said, "Because of my physical condition, I don't believe this virus is going to overtake me. People with this attitude have survived and are looking good." Here he makes an assumption about causality. People may have done well for purely biologic reasons (e.g., having a less powerful strain), though he and others then seek psychological explanations to account for the success.

Roger assumes that his comparative good health until now predicts a good outcome. "I've had the virus for nine years. If I made it this far, there is no reason why I can't make it for another nine years. Why should anything change now? People look at my palm and tell me I have a long lifeline. I trust that more than the fact that I'm HIV positive." He and others thus seek evidence elsewhere to support their minimization. Although some people have remained "only HIV positive," researchers still insist that all HIV will eventually lead to AIDS. Yet the fact that some people appear to progress slowly, if at all, offers hope to others.

Reynaldo Fernandez, who had had a nightmare about being on an AIDS ward, goes even further in trying to forget he even has HIV. "Sometimes I forget that I'm HIV. I try to get my head blank. I don't want to start thinking too much about certain issues and start going overboard on them. I try to keep some things out of my thoughts. This weekend I could have gone to a couple of AIDS meetings, but I stayed home. I just didn't feel like going. The weather wasn't great. Some friends' houses have literature all over the place. Everything says AIDS and HIV. But home is supposed to be a place where you're comfortable and can relax and get rid of stress. I try to live like I don't have HIV. I go out and forget it.

"I try to keep my mind busy so that the thought won't bother me. I'll run around doing something else. I meditate and do breathing exercises, trying to keep thoughts out of my head. Going to the hospital and dealing with dead people is the worst thing people could do. I read spy thrillers. They help me keep my thoughts away from some of the things going on around me. I get lost in the books. They're a good way to escape from a lot of things." Reynaldo avoids HIV, yet he also feels "something's missing in my life," and his dream reveals that his illness remains with him, even if unconsciously.

Positive attitudes can clearly verge on denial. As Jenny Singer said, "I don't want to change my life to revolve around the disease completely, so I try not to dwell on it. My husband likes to talk about it a lot more than I do. I try to change the subject. I just kind of turn my mind off, or put the TV on, even if I'm not watching. I could be just staring into space, but the noise helps distract me. Or I start cleaning around the house or doing something in the back-yard. I wake up every day thinking this day may be my last. I'm grateful for every day I have. Yet I could also get hit by a car today or get mugged. Anything can happen. I don't believe I'm going to die from AIDS. I feel I'm going to fight it. I have a very positive at-titude that it's not going to get me. I keep telling myself that I'm not going to get sick. Maybe it's denial, maybe I'm not looking at things realistically. I may be fooling myself. I don't know."

Yet reality intrudes. "Sometimes I do have doubts. The other day I saw Kimberly Bergalis on TV. Her arms were skinny. They were spoon-feeding her—that knocked me hard and brought the reality home to me. It makes me wonder if I am denying I have the virus by saying, 'I'm not going to get sick like her.' " Jenny thus tries to deny not that she has the virus but that it will progress.

"I'm the kind of person that has to see to believe, and I don't see or feel it. It isn't in my mind that I'm dying. I say I'm going to overcome this. I don't consider that denial because I'm very aware of what I'm dealing with. I'm not saying I don't have HIV. I've been diagnosed with AIDS and ARC. But just because I've had PCP, TB, and shingles, and get fatigued, doesn't make me 'a girl with AIDS' "—that is, that the illness is defining, an identity. "I refuse to feel that. If that's denial, I like it. I don't want to walk around feeling miserable all the time, and I think that's a way of dealing with it and giving it a good fight. Patients on TV can't walk, lose their balance, their hair, their nails, their weight, and their color. It could happen. But I don't feel it, so it's not there. I'll deal with it when I see it."

For Alfie Montoya too, "positive thinking" can have potentially dangerous countereffects. "I'm not going anywhere," he said. "I don't look at myself as dying anytime soon. I'm thirty-seven and have a lot of life ahead of me. I tell everyone that they're invited to my one hundredth birthday. I'll lick this," he continues, as if the virus can be vanquished. His belief parallels that of the basketball star Magic Johnson, who announced in words that became a headline, "I'll beat the virus," as if it were a sports opponent, and a beatable one at that. Alfie Montoya goes on, "Most people treat me as if nothing was wrong, and that's because of the way I carry myself. I don't talk sick, look sick, act sick, or walk around sick; so other people don't look at me that way either. I'm 'living with AIDS' because the doctor told me I had AIDS. But I don't feel it. I've never felt better. I'm off drugs now, take better care of myself, and am in touch with my family again. I had some illnesses but don't have them today, so I don't worry whether I'm going to get sick." Unfortunately Alfie soon returned to drugs, perhaps thinking too positively and not "talking sick" enough.

Positive thinking about HIV can thus be naive. Denial has never been as deadly, since those who deny HIV may be more likely to spread it to others through unsafe sex or needle sharing.

Yet denial means different things to different people. The term's popular usage extends beyond its psychoanalytic definition as a defense mechanism, but in both senses it implies pathology and carries a negative connotation. Those said to be "in denial" are derided for their blindness toward themselves, their lack of self-knowledge and self-awareness. A culture that places its highest philosophical value on knowing oneself looks askance at deficient self-knowledge.

Still, many use the term when speaking about themselves. Denial becomes a place definable, with protected borders. As Jill Montgomery said, "I came out of denial almost two and a half years ago. I didn't want to deal with HIV. So it wasn't there. Then I came into sobriety"—also in many ways a place.

These distinctions become important. The psychiatrist George Valliant has categorized defenses by their level of maturity, and he ranks "suppression"—being aware of a problem but choosing not to focus on it—as one of the highest. In contrast he ranks "repression"—not being conscious of an impulse or problem—and denial itself much lower.

"I practice conscious denial," Leonard Barber said. "I pretend I'm going to live forever, even though I know I'm not. It's a game, no more real than playing Monopoly, but it's the only way that makes sense to me. In the beginning I thought, 'Oh my God, I can't commit myself to anything that takes more than a year because I could be sick in bed.' That doesn't seem to me now to be a very useful approach. The only way for me to have a life at all is to make decisions as though nothing is wrong with me and I'm going to live forever—like everybody thinks they are. I'm not going to let go of parts of my life until I have to. I see no reason to foreclose options that will inevitably happen—HIV or not—because of aging. Everything would be completely meaningless and absurd. Nobody really believes in their own mortality.

"I'd be surprised if I were dead in a year, but it's not an impossibility. It would also be surprising if I'm not dead in ten or fifteen years. But if I were to start doing the things that people do when they think they've only got a year to go, and then it turns out that I live, I'll just have lived perversely. If I assume I don't have a future at all, I would just stop living." Perhaps because of these beliefs, Leonard concentrates on gardening—planting trees and bushes that will survive him.

All I Want: Bargaining

"Bargaining" can provide a reasonable if fragile degree of certainty and control over unpredictability and the threat of annihilation, a trouble-free if time-limited future. Calvin Taylor, a thirty-five-year-old African-American man with a history of injecting drug use, now lives in an AIDS residence. "I don't want to live fifteen or twenty years," he told me. "Two or three years is fine for me. I pray to God that he just gives me enough time to go home to Georgia. But whatever he gives me, I'm all right with. I don't care about blood transfusions or anything like that.

"I'm not looking forward to dying, but I'm gonna die because I got full-blown AIDS. I have to accept that. I'm not scared of death. I'm ready for it.

"I'm tired. All my life I've been running, going to this city and that, and I've been through two or three women, traveling. I never did sit and stay. That's what I want to do now. Down South I can get a little cheap house with two acres. I could see the peaches come out, walk down the road, smell the cow shit, hunt for deer. I used to do that. But I became a dope fiend for twenty years and got away from it. Now I just want to live and die like that. That would make me happy.

"In high school I played football and basketball, but then I got into trouble because of drugs. I started drinking when I was fourteen. My father and my mom both died of cirrhosis of the liver. My granddad, my uncle, and about fifteen people in my family drink. I come from a history of drinking. I thought I was supposed to drink. My parents fought every weekend. Friday they got paid, Friday and Saturday night they fought. They went to church Sunday and to the factory Monday. That happened my whole time growing up. My father wasn't a role model. He drank a lot.

"My football coach *was* a role model. He kept me in school and got me a job in a youth program, working during the summer. He took me shopping for shoes and clothes. I played good ball. He came from a poor neighborhood too, so he knew what was going on. He would come by my house and talk to my mom. Once when I got in trouble drinking, he gave me a talking to. He wanted me to go to college. I was good enough to go, he told my mother. No one in my family had ever gone to college. But I got into trouble stealing and had to do nine months. When I came back I went to

Georgia Tech to study food management, but drugs caught up with me and I dropped out.

"I never did big time in jail, and jail never filled me with fear because I wasn't scared of nothing. I've always been a good fighter.

"But I feel guilty because I was a good athlete and wanted to be a college coach. I could have been. I had the opportunity. I was one of the best boxers, and I boxed in the state tournament. In '80 I boxed in the Olympic trials. I did a little coaching and learned how to handle kids too. But dope took a lot out of me. There's a lot of things I wish I did.

"When I was using, if I had a TV I'd sell it. I used to get $99 every two weeks from welfare, and I'd shoot it all up. One time I bought a phone, and the next day I went out and sold it to buy drugs. It wasn't until later I thought that was stupid. I was lonely and drugs made me who I wanted to be—slick and without problems.

"But I can't pick up now. I want to die sober. I don't want to die sick. I've been real sick. One time I had to wear a diaper. I just want to lay down now. I enjoy myself being in here because I can shut the door and take the phone off the hook. I ain't got to be bothered by nobody. I can call downstairs and say that I don't want any visitors.

"Now, here in my room I got cable and many channels. I can get a VCR if I want. I go on trips. People call me for help. I have ten pairs of shoes that people donated.

"Sometimes I go up on the roof and look out by myself. I look at the river and the way the water flows and think about my home in Georgia. I used to go fishing. I just dream and feel good up there, all right with the world. Then I come down here by myself and read the Bible or the paper.

"Everybody's got how and where they want to die. I want to die on my own soil. I don't want to die in New York. I'm old-fashioned. I want to be buried with my parents in the graveyard along with my older brother, my aunt, my grandma and granddad. If I die here, my soul wouldn't be satisfied. My spirit would never rest.

"I believe in spirits; I dream about my mama and my brother all the time. I want to die and be with them. The Bible says God is a good God, righteous. I don't think he'll make me suffer twice. This is hell. Probably when you die you go to a place and rest. Your soul goes to judgment. If you do what he told you, you go to the Promised Land where there's no pain or sickness.

"Dying in Georgia will give me insurance. When someone dies, I think I might be next and haven't done what I want: gone home. Lord have mercy if I have to die here. I just want to see home one more time. I'm doing the necessary things. I'm not an angel, but I go to the hospital to visit people. I'm doing that for the Lord and for me. He judges everybody on a different standard. Everybody can't pray the same way. Some people pray with big words. I just talk to him. That's all I do.

"I have no fear about death. My biggest fear is picking up. If I hadn't gone to the program and come here, I'd still be fucked up."

"I've been off drugs for two and a half years now, but every day I still get a powerful urge to use them and have to pick up the phone and talk to friends—sometimes for two or three hours—until the urge passes. I think I can do that for two or three more years, but not fifteen or twenty years. I don't want to take no chances. If I lived longer than two or three years, I'd probably go back to drugs. And I want to die clean."

The problem with this kind of bargaining is what to do when the self-allotted period of time passes and one is still alive. Elsa Diaz, now living with her grown daughter, solves this problem by "giving myself six months at a time. If nothing happens within six months, I add another six months to live. I do this because every time I hear somebody has died, they got the results of the test six months earlier. I've also seen people that had the virus and in six months were just eaten up by it. So I say every six months I'll see what happens. I look for any changes: did I lose any weight, am I losing my memory or speaking slow? I look for any difference in my face—skin rashes and scars. It's been a few years but I still do that."

Drug users in particular often had developed their own notions of time and the future even before HIV. As Arlene Chambers explains, "I was never one of those people that said, 'Oh, I'll take a trip in six months.' I can't do that. I have to plan it out one month at a time. I've planned things longer but they never turned out. I hope I'm one of the fortunate persons who will be helped when they find a cure. But it's like hitting the lottery."

Gloria Higgens said, "I might get sick next month. It might be ten years. Who knows? I just take one day at a time." This sort of AA approach helps to deal with stresses arising from the uncertainty of the prognosis.

The blocks of time sought vary in length. As Gloria adds, "My new boyfriend and I decided to give ourselves time periods of ten years. For the next ten years we're gonna be all right and not think about it. We've agreed that for ten years we're just going to exist. No matter what happens we're just going to be there together and live and have fun like normal people. After that we don't know. It sounds like a good amount of time. In ten years maybe I'll get to see a grandchild. We'll think about another time limit once those ten years come and go."

Whom Gloria and others bargain with remains unclear—presumably God. But these men and women balance internal desires with an assumed external moral force. Such bargaining implicitly affirms the existence of a higher power that influences destiny. Yet an inner sense of equity and justice dictates the exact terms of these agreements. These men and woman permit themselves a degree of liberty in exchange for longer-term survival. Thus this mode of minimization, as with others, allows for a sense of "normalcy," freedom from the virus's effects, at least for a time.

Minimization thus assumes various forms and degrees. Denial, though meaning different things to different people, arises here in multiple guises. For example, the "positive" stance toward HIV adopted by many can itself verge on minimization. Aspects of the illness and individuals' own backgrounds contribute to such responses, and men and women employ a range of strategies. Yet these "positive" approaches to HIV can predispose to problems, including substance abuse and unsafe sex. Thus minimization, while reducing the threat and dread of HIV, can ultimately impair health.

NINE

Free Like a Bird:
Drugs and HIV

ALCOHOL AND DRUGS also provide momentary escape from the "shame," anxiety, and despair of HIV. Drugs are intricately tied to HIV: injection drug use constitutes the fastest-growing source of infection. Addiction can cause chaos, ruling and ruining lives, and leading to indifference to one's own health and that of others. Drug use can seem intractable, yet HIV can also prompt sobriety and the adoption of more effective means of coping.

All I Thought About

Jill Montgomery, who now lives in a "house of positive people," said, "When I first found out I was infected, I had that 'Fuck it' attitude. HIV was a hassle. I didn't care. I was dying—so what? I started using even heavier to get away from it.

"I was suffering but didn't want anybody to know. I tried to cover it all up and make it all nice with drugs. I was hoping I would die and get it over with. Nobody really knew who Jill was, what made Jill tick. They couldn't understand why I always eventually went back into drugs. But I couldn't deal with pressure. All I ever thought about was where my bag of dope would come from. I didn't care what I had to do to get it, who I had to rob, as long as I got high. Drugs made me feel free like a bird. No responsibility, no problems—a beautiful feeling. What came afterward I didn't like—sleeping two or three days and getting up and going into the same cycle over and over and over.

"I was living in the streets, in abandoned buildings, not knowing where my next meal was coming from. I ran a shooting gallery. My father's a diabetic, and he used to bring me syringes to sell. I supported my habit by hitting people's veins. A lot of people couldn't inject themselves, so I would. They paid me in money or drugs.

"I'd be there for two or three days, then sleep two or three days. Sometimes I didn't know what day or month it was. Spring, summer, winter—it was all the same to me. I got ear infections. My asthma came back. I would be in the hospital two weeks, then on the street for two months, then wind up back in the hospital for another two weeks. My weight went from 135 to 96 pounds. I thought, 'Fuck, I'm going to die. Let everyone else die too.' All I cared about was dope. People said HIV was around, but I didn't care. I figured, 'What the hell? I'm going to die anyway.'

"When I'm using drugs they're my main concern. I might think I gotta do this or that, but I can't because my main concern is dope; it takes me over completely. Sometimes I'd get money and say, 'I'm gonna go see my daughter and get her sneakers.' I might even get halfway there, but then I'd turn around. I used to joke, 'I'll die with a spike in my arm, high, and won't feel a thing.' When I'm 'sick'—that is, in withdrawal—all I think about is getting straight. And if there's only one syringe, I'll share it. I'll rinse it out and use it. That's just how it is. I'm not going to think about getting two dollars and buying a new one. Just get the drugs into my system to feel well again. I didn't have no alternative.

"I was doing anything and everything that would get me high, put me to sleep, make me forget. I would feel happy, but really I was miserable. I couldn't talk to anybody; nobody really cared. I was hurting my family a lot but didn't want to face them. There wasn't one night I didn't cry or think about them. But I was scared. I thought they would reject me, so I didn't see them. At one point my son went around saying I was already dead. He didn't want to talk to me. I can't blame him. He feels I neglected and abandoned him, which I did. I wasn't around for two or three years. I left my mother in charge. My eight-year-old daughter does not know I'm her mother. My five-year-old thinks I'm his cousin or aunt. My nine-year-old daughter knows that I'm her mother but says, 'You're the mother that brought me into this world. But that's my real mother.' With a nine-year-old, you can't really push it that much.

"I lost a lot of friends. Some didn't want to bother with me because of my drugs. At one time I had good friends, but they pushed away from me.

"People who hadn't seen me in a while would say, 'Wow! You're still around? I heard you were dead.' I'd say, 'Yeah, I'm still around. I haven't died yet. No, I'm not dead.'

"But I was giving up everything. There was no place to go. I would get up every morning and say, 'God, how much longer do I have?' I found myself praying to Jesus, saying, 'I don't want to die like this.' I wanted to see my kids and be able to see grandkids. My oldest daughter is in college, but I don't know where. I know she graduated from high school in Brooklyn.

"I went into the hospital again, this time for two months. A social worker there told me, 'Jill, if you go back to the streets you're not going to be here next year.' I couldn't walk, and they were going to cut off my leg. I was riding in a wheelchair. I had suffered so much in life, I didn't want to go like this—another one dying in an abandoned building and put in a plastic bag. She told me about this place, a shelter that would only be temporary. I'm still there. I know I can't do drugs now, because one is never enough and a thousand's too many."

Garbage Head

Drug use can become deeply entrenched, part of an identity. Barriers to the use of drugs can fall despite awareness of potential medical complications.

"I was a dope fiend and still am," Donny Sotelo told me. "I'll be one until I die." A twenty-six-year-old Latino, he is tall and outgoing. He met me wearing a red, white, and blue windbreaker, the sleeves rolled up, and sat with his leg swung up on a chair near him, casual and relaxed. "When I sit around doing nothing, out of the blue I'll think, 'Oh boy, ho hum, let me go get a bag or smoke crack.' And I'll stay out there. I'll look up and it's two days later. I'll be out in the streets stealing, selling, or being a lookout."

"Every day I want to get high. But the day I tested positive, the urge to get high went from a little feeling to filling up the whole room and pushed me out the door. I walked out. I had been there with some guys and walked right past them. They asked what's wrong and I said, 'Nothing. I got to go home.' But in the back of my mind I was saying, 'Let me go back to the streets.' That was on Friday. On Sunday morning I woke up and looked out the window. I must have slept two hours in three days.

"I've been arrested eight times, seven of them for drugs. No matter what garbage it is—speedballs, crack—if it's there, I'll do it. I'm a garbage head. I say to myself, 'It's a small thing, only $5, go ahead.' I say 'Later' for everything. I hustled. I think now about scams I pulled. I was using $150 worth of drugs every day. If someone got me mad, instead of me dealing with the person over whatever it was, I would go out and shoot a bag of dope or smoke crack.

"Call it dope-fiend rationale. I said, 'My T-cell count is high, I can afford to kill T-cells. My general health is not bad.' I rationalized it was okay to relapse.

"I still dream about drugs—that I'm down in the Lower East Side where I used to buy them. The other night I dreamed I was in an abandoned building. When I was out there in real life I was dirty and didn't shower or change my clothes. But in the dream I was clean. I was scraping the cooker, trying to get a last shot. When an addict's finished drugging and doesn't have any more drugs, there's a little bit left in the cooker—the cap—and you add a little water and scrape it. Sometimes I'll be shooting up nothing but water because almost no drug is left. But in the dreams something always happens and I never get high. I wake up or the syringe breaks.

"I should put money aside to take a nice trip—a reward to myself for being good, taking care of myself, doing the right thing. But when I get the money I spend it to get high. I rationalize: why shouldn't I enjoy myself? I deserve to get high once in a while. If I'm going to die soon, why shouldn't I enjoy the last few years of my life?

"I've also felt a little sorry for myself, I guess. Depressed. Blue. Drugs help me forget."

His drug use increases in part because HIV triggers regret about his life. "I was always the black sheep," Donny continues. "I goofed up my life. I could have had a profession. But I was too busy hanging out in the street, being cool instead of square. The squares now are the ones enjoying life. My nephew is now an assistant bank manager and goes to the Bahamas and is hip. I'm a square now because I can't do anything. I wasted my life.

"I wasn't stupid. One teacher wrote on a report card that I had the makings of a good student if I'd just stay in class longer. My mother says I should have been a lawyer or a doctor because I did really well in school. I was a B-plus student. I think about the things I blew. I managed a store once. My brother-in-law said, 'I wish I had half the shit you had: girls, girls with cars. One of the girls you were supposed to stay with had a house, two cars, and a nice job. You could've been living lovely with her instead of living in the fucking street. I did drugs just like you but I functioned and went to work. All you did was work and shoot dope.' I told him, 'If you were somebody else, I would punch you in your face.'

"I just never finished things I started. I went to computer school for a six-month course and dropped out after four months. I was the number two student in the class. I was going to an eight-week course in AIDS intervention and dropped out after five weeks. I went to college and dropped out after two years. I went to high school, dropped out, went back, dropped out again, went into the military, stayed for a year, and got thrown out. People say, 'You could be sitting behind a desk or standing in front of a classroom.' I have the potential, the personality. I got something I can share and a lot of people could benefit from. But I'm a day-to-day type of person. I don't look way down the road—maybe one block, two blocks ahead."

"I saw my ex-girlfriend who said, 'You know, you are really a great person. I don't know why you don't look past tomorrow.' I thought, 'What the fuck do I got for tomorrow?' Now I know what.

"I feel bad I'm not living up to my potential. They say a hard head makes a soft behind: you pay the consequences of being hardheaded instead of listening. I knew that going to shooting galleries and having sex with all these girls might give me HIV. But I did it; I can't do nothing to change it now." Still he relapses, potentially impairing his immune system even further. Sadly and ironically, his regrets about using drugs prompt him to use more drugs.

"But I do try to help others learn from my mistakes. In college, before I dropped out, I wanted to be a teacher. So it's funny because now I get to educate people. What I learn I pass on to the next person. I want people to know, to understand. I try to spread the word, not the virus. I'm a savior in that things come to me and I put them back together for the next guy. If I can share what I learned, I feel good now."

Born to Be a Junkie and Die

In the world of drugs, even the threat of death—from HIV or another drug-related problem—often fails to motivate abstinence. Instead death becomes seen as inevitable. As Alfie Montoya explained, "I always said I'm not gonna live past thirty-five anyway, because I was that wild, always getting into trouble, being in the wrong places, dealing with people that normal people wouldn't deal with, like drug suppliers. I was always running. I used to hang out with street gangs, motorcycle gangs. When the cops pulled me over I'd say, 'What's wrong, officer?' A lot of the cops knew me. I thought it was a matter of time until I died. So I thought I'd go out the way I knew best: using drugs. I sent myself out on a mission, a rampage, trying to commit suicide with drugs. I lived in an abandoned building. In the daytime I used all the money I made the night before. During the night I stayed up, working in drug spots or selling works. Or if I couldn't, I would hustle, panhandle. I started stealing, breaking into factories. I used drugs even more heavily than before HIV. I used to use one bundle of dope a day, then I started three, four, or five bundles. I began a drug rehab program but had no intentions of stopping. Using drugs was all I knew how to do. In the rehab I was supposed to be learning how to deal with life, but life was turning on me. At the time a person with AIDS was believed to have a year to eighteen months to live. AIDS equaled death. I had been sentenced to die! I thought, 'What the hell am I doing in a program?' Let me just go out and shoot all the drugs I could find. I might as well enjoy the last few weeks or months I had. I cursed the world out. I felt the world owed me something. I didn't know what.

"I started using drugs at the age of nine. I grew up poor in the Lower East Side. My father was an alcoholic and my mother didn't speak English, so she couldn't get a job. I dropped out of eighth grade and started using drugs because they made me feel like the person I wanted to be—outspoken. I was shy. Drugs made me able to talk, rap to girls, hang out. I didn't think about my problems. I also liked the money. That was a big part of it. I started shooting up when I was sixteen.

"I've contracted many diseases in my life because of drugs: gonorrhea, syphilis, herpes. You name it, I've had it—every drug-caused disease there is. I was convinced I was born to be a junkie and die." Fate here blends probability and morality, the results of economics and background.

"I figured that since I was going to die, let me die high. When I'm stoned I don't think about nothing. When I'm not stoned I chase bags, trying to get stoned. Dope is a bad medicine because you can get pains in your body and can't walk. But it's good for the mind because you forget all your problems. When I feel down, I just want to get high. I figure that will help me."

Denial plays an important role in this drug world. "I forgot I was HIV. I didn't think about it. When I got to the detox the health counselor asked me if I had gotten tested for the virus. I told her yes. She said, 'Would you like to tell us the results?' I said, 'It came back negative,' though I knew it was positive. She asked me how long ago that was. I told her seven, eight months. She said, 'Would you like to take the test again?' That's what I wanted her to say, because I was hoping that if I took the test again it would come back negative. So I went. The detox sent two people with me for support. When I came out of the office after getting the results, I put on a big, phony smile. They asked me, 'What happened? Are you all right?' I told them, 'Yeah, man! It came back negative. I'm glad. I wouldn't want to deal with this.'

"When I got back to the detox, the health counselor asked me if I cared to talk to her or share the results. And I told her, 'Yeah.' She asked, 'How did it go?' I said, 'Great! It came back negative.' She said, 'That's good.' Then she asked, 'You got a minute?' I said, 'Yeah.' And she said, 'You know, you remind me of a resident that was here about five months ago.' I said, 'Why? Do you think I'm related to him or something?' She said, 'No, no it's nothing like that. But when he got his results—for one reason or another, the way you're acting and the impression you're giving me remind me of him. He came back and acted exactly like you and said he was negative. Two days later he split and started getting high, and it turned out he had tested positive but couldn't deal with it. Now I would just hate to see that happen to you. I'm not saying you're lying to me, I'm just saying what I'm feeling and what I see. If it's like you say, I'm really glad for you. But if it's not, whenever you want to talk, we can.' She was knocking down all my defenses. I thought about whether to tell her and finally said, 'You're right. I was positive even before I came here,' and I explained that I didn't want the others to know because I thought they would back away from me. I've been very alone in my life, and thought people wouldn't want to be in the same room or sleep near me. If the staff knew, I was pretty sure the residents would too." It's interesting that Alfie's deception here mirrors his earlier description of the virus itself as slick and able to disguise itself.

"When I was out there, I didn't have any fears of the virus. I thought if I snorted, I wouldn't catch AIDS. Being clean is nice, but deep inside I always want to get high. I might get that 'I don't care' syndrome. That's what got me here in the first place. I got tired and just gave up on a lot of things. It's a difficult world. Addiction is a monster. HIV's a monster too, but not as much. You don't go through withdrawal pains like with addiction. HIV doesn't attack you all at once. One time a guy was panicking because his needle clogged up, and he offered me ten dollars for my set. I told him it was used and that I was sick. He said, 'I don't care. Here's ten dollars.' So I gave him the needle. I got ten dollars for more drugs, and I had warned him. It was his choice. He bought himself HIV. He was sick, withdrawing, needed a fix, and wasn't thinking. The only thing in his mind was getting the drug in his body. When you're withdrawing, and all hyper, nothing else matters. I also learned in the street that there are no friends."

Addiction maintains a tight grip. "Right now the only thing keeping me from using is HIV. But if they ever came up with a cure, I'd probably go back to drugs."

Where Numbness Stops Being Numb

Escape from this land of drugs can seem impossible. As Beatrice Rosaro, who now has grandchildren, described it, "One night, very late, I was standing on the corner and couldn't move. My stomach felt like somebody had kicked it in. My boyfriend at the time had a constant pain in the chest, a cough, thinness, and night sweats. And because we were active heroin addicts, we ignored these things. It was raining and I was dirty because he was dragging me all over. That's when I decided I had had enough. I said to my boyfriend, 'Let's take a cab to the hospital.' He had a couple of dollars, but no cab would stop. That's how bad we looked. Somehow, though, we got to the hospital. I don't remember if we walked or if a cab finally took us. I fainted right on the emergency room floor. I was skinny and had pneumonia and was dying. The doctor came later and said, 'I have news to tell you about the test we've taken. You have AIDS.' I was stunned and cried for the whole day. The first thing I thought about was my family. How's my mother and my son gonna take this? I signed myself out of the hospital and got sedated. I didn't want to think about it or tell anybody." For Beatrice and many others, drug use initially increases rather than declines after a positive HIV test.

In a culture of poverty, drug use also becomes part of a vicious cycle. "My mother had five kids out of wedlock. Then my father left her, messed around, and had four children with another woman and lived on the same block as us. My poor mother had to work to support five children. It was terrible. My brother in high school had holes in the bottom of his shoes, and he went to my father to ask for fifty cents for the shoe repair. My father said he didn't have the money, and then went downstairs and came back up with a six-pack of beer. We'd go over there and his other daughters all had dolls and pretty pink stuff and bureaus full of Avon stuff for little girls, and pretty clothes and shoes in the closet, while we had to do with what we had.

"On Father's Day this year I finally decided to call my dad and say, 'Happy Father's Day.' He said, 'Oh, thank you,' and then started: 'Now is when you call. You never bother to throw your father ten dollars.' I love my father. I do not hate him. And I understand that he's a sick person—he has the disease of alcoholism, and cancer of the esophagus and the stomach from the alcoholism. Half his stomach is gone. He has a plastic tube. But he's drinking again. And I'm angry about it. That's why I hadn't called him. I said, 'Well, at least I called now.' That was it. I got it over with."

Drugs offered her escape. "I wanted to be numb all the time and not feel the pain of life—remembering my childhood, my three failed marriages, and my husband who was beating me, losing my family and my children, not having a home, sleeping on park benches, and going to jail. I wanted to feel nothing, to exist without feeling. I could still feel, but I started not to care and made up my mind that all of this was unimportant. All I was doing day and night was getting high, and on top of that, getting beaten up constantly.

"If I had $500, it was gone in an hour. That's a lot of drugs. You can't get any more numb. And then I'd be at the point of numbness where numbness stops being numb, and feelings just start seeping through. If you turn the water on and hold the faucet, the pressure goes up until you can't hold it no more and the water spills through.

"Using drugs, I didn't think much about the future, just about getting my next bag, my next fix. I thought, 'How can I live without a drug?' I knew drugs were bad for me, but I still used them. I'd wasted my life anyway." Her goal now is to stay clean for her grandchildren.

For Beatrice and other women, drug use often appears somewhat forced upon them, rather than sought out as it is with some of the men. Olana, Gerry, and Carrie, for example, still exude warmth and genuine concern for their children—often abandoned by fathers—and others. Carol Gilligan, a Harvard psychologist, in her book *In a Different Voice,* has written that women differ from men in following a concern for others, rather than abstract principles, as the basis for a moral life. These women frequently had few options or resources for coping with the enormous stresses of poverty and urban decay.

Yet the effects of drugs can be overpowering. In fact, addiction—more than homosexuality—shapes the lives of those gay men who also abuse substances. In many ways these men, in their desperation and sacrifice of all else for drugs, resemble other addicts more than other gay men.

Last Chances

Among some men and women, HIV can motivate abstinence. Elsa Diaz, living with her grown daughter, said, "The doctor told me I'd be dead in six months if I didn't give up drugs. I didn't want to speed the virus up. I stopped because I knew that otherwise I would die. If I had another bag, it would be my last. I was sick and saw everyone around me dying. It took HIV to get me to stop." That she didn't see drugs but only HIV as threatening her life surprised me.

Twelve-step programs such as AA, NA (Narcotics Anonymous), and CA (Cocaine Anonymous) can help people quit and remain sober. Positives Anonymous, an HIV-positive twelve-step program, and specific gay HIV-positive AA groups have also developed.

Drug use and HIV interact in several ways. As Donny Sotelo explained, "I have two diseases—addiction and the virus. If I forget I'm an addict and focus totally on the disease, I'll end up using drugs. If I focus too much on my addiction, I'll forget I have the virus. So I make meetings for both. On Fridays I go to NA and PA—Positives Anonymous—which talks about the virus, not drugs." But by themselves these programs are often not enough. As Alfie Montoya said, "I met a guy, clean twenty years, who relapsed. I have to fight this shit hard and long for the rest of my life. My only goal now is staying clean and maintaining my health. Every time I want to stop fighting, I think, 'No man, that's not going to work.' I think about weighing 135 pounds, being smoked out, having tracks all over me, being thin, dirty, stinking, and scruffy. I ain't going there again."

Stopping drugs can nevertheless be transforming. "HIV was a blessing in disguise," Gregory Colson said, "a second chance. I'm not sick now. I'm more healthy than two years ago. I've gained weight. My whole life has changed for the better. My family is very happy, especially my mother because she has me back in her life after twenty-seven years of drugs. They had lost me. I didn't visit them. All I did was just live for drugs. I used drugs and they used me. Nothing else mattered. I wasn't living. There was no life: I didn't go to movies or date or have sex."

Olana Ramirez says AIDS "gave me a chance to be a human again. I recently dreamed of saving my daughter from drowning in a boat. I reached out and grabbed her out of the water and into the dry boat." Yet it seems here as if she was saving herself too. Using drugs is viewed as analogous to being dead or near dead; being free of drugs is being alive, at least in terms of the overall effect on daily life and functioning. Yet, as she adds, "It's a shame that it took HIV for me to realize I could like myself off drugs."

Relapses of drug use continue even among the most fervent abstainers, often spurred on by HIV-related stresses. Donny confessed, "I was clean for two years until I got sick from HIV. Then I picked up again. I thought I could use drugs once in a while. It was bullshit. Here I was, a drug counselor, teaching other people not to use drugs, and I started to use myself. I lost my girlfriend—if both people in a relationship use drugs, there is no relationship. It's not love. You become drug partners, and addicts are very selfish, greedy, inconsiderate, and uncaring. My world just crumbled in."

To feel empathy for these men and women can be difficult. Yet they too are patients—suffering and struggling, often to rid themselves of addiction. Drug use can join with poverty in a vicious cycle from which escape appears impossible. But many of these individuals, prompted by the virus, are able to abstain and turn their lives around. Understanding their lives and their world can reveal the obstacles to and the possible ways of reducing the epidemic's further spread. The continued pursuit of drugs, despite health risks, suggests the extent of the stress and pain HIV creates.

Part III: IMPLICATIONS

TEN

Caving In: *Anxiety and Despair*

HAVING ILLUSTRATED the six broad patterns of handling the stresses of HIV, we can see they have critical psychological and medical implications. All these patterns are responses to losses and the sense of taboo resulting from the illness; they provide ways of managing such rejection and widespread death. Four of these modes of response—immersion in HIV-land, appeal to higher powers, work and volunteerism, and increasing ties with family—also provide important sources of meaning and symbolic immortality which can help buffer the depression, anxiety, and "existential angst" resulting from the infection. A fifth pattern, minimization of the illness, can also alleviate psychological symptoms, though other problems of health behavior may result. The sixth response, substance use, may numb painful feelings fleetingly but contribute in the long run to other difficulties.

Individuals follow these patterns in distinctive ways. Among former injecting drug users, for example, Gregory Colson and Gerry Galvez found hope through spirituality and volunteerism, while Carrie Serano and Elsa Diaz looked to their families. Alfie

Montoya minimized the illness, felt better for a period of time, but eventually returned to drugs, potentially spreading the virus to others. Among gay men, George Sullivan, outgoing and gregarious, participated in HIV-land; Jason Gillian, quieter and more reserved, became even more religious. Ken Landers, who felt he had little to show for his life, having failed as an actor, minimized the impact of the illness on his life and dreams. Leonard Barber, having lived in the country for several years, turned to nature. Individuals thus acted because of social or personal reasons, and sometimes changed strategies over time as a result of medical, social, and psychological events.

Those patients who said they "felt positive" about "being positive" in fact followed one or more of these six patterns. Usually one such pattern predominated. Yet patients didn't attribute their acceptance of the virus to their adoption of these patterns. Wilma, for example, didn't say the virus ceased to bother her *because* she was "born again." Rather, she said she now accepted the virus and later discussed her newfound spirituality. Similarly Ken didn't say the virus disturbed him *because* he minimized it. These patterns of response provide solace in ways not always apparent to the patients themselves—unconsciously as well as consciously.

Again and again in these narratives, themes of death and rebirth arose, whether socially ("a new community"), theologically ("a new age"), biologically ("a new generation"), or professionally ("a new career"), or conversely through resistance and minimization ("I'm still the old me, unchanged"). The construction of a new world in these ways attempts to resolve problems resulting from rejection and death.

Final Solutions: Thinking About Suicide

In the absence of any of these response patterns, depression and despair as well as suicidal thoughts more commonly occur. Raoul Rodriquez, having moved to this country from Mexico, was raised Catholic but recently has had religious doubts. "I feel lonely, hopeless, and depressed," he told me in the small apartment he shares with his sister and her husband. "My life is a failure. What is the purpose of this fucking life anyway? My family looked up to me as a model, as a hero for having come here to America. Now all I have to show for it is this virus. Sometimes I have thoughts of suicide. I want to solve all this bullshit and find peace. I had never considered suicide before. But a few times since HIV, I've thought of doing something. I keep those thoughts to myself as a final solution and haven't discussed them with my therapist." Raoul, uncomfortable in America, avoids HIV-land. He attended a support group a few times but dropped out. He also missed the last several sessions with his therapist, whom he sees at a gay mental health clinic.

At my first meeting with him I persuaded him to go again to his support group and his therapist. When I next saw him, he had done both. "I've begun to feel better—a lot more optimistic, even at work, just like in the old days."

Depression and anxiety occur more commonly in association with alcohol and drug use. As Eddie Lourdes, who now feels he has a "second chance," explained, "Two years ago in January I was disgusted with the way I was living. One Sunday I had no money and managed to get some needles to sell. But it took a long time to unload them. At three in the morning it was freezing outside. I was cold and wished I were dead. Finally I got ten dollars and bought a bag of coke. But then a guy came up to me and put a gun to my head to mug me for the cocaine. I looked at him and said, 'Do me a favor and pull the goddam trigger. I'm dying any-way.' He stood there dumbfounded. I turned and walked away, expecting him to shoot me in the back of my head, but he didn't. I looked up to the sky and cursed God: 'You ain't shit, you know? What are you doing, leaving me down here suffering? Why don't you hurry up and let this virus eat me away, or let me overdose and die?' I went home and shot the coke." He gave up drugs shortly thereafter.

Realistic views of their illness, in the absence of any of these pat-terns of adaptation, can also lead to depression. For example, Kerry Musgrove is not religious, doesn't minimize his illness, and is estranged from his family. As a paid volunteer in an AIDS orga-nization, he struggles to help others dying from the same disease. He tries to think positively, but that alone isn't enough. "I've been one of the lucky people. When I was diagnosed I never thought I would be here five years later. I had a dozen KS lesions, a month later a dozen more, and the month after that even more. I thought, 'In another year I'm going to be ready to kill myself because I'm not going to walk around covered with ten thousand lesions.' But then they stopped. I realized it wasn't as bad as it first seemed. Early last year I painted my apartment. I thought that was a good sign. It meant I believed life could go on. I had to do things, not to last twenty-five years—it would have to be painted again some time—but at least I could accomplish short-term goals. I could improve things around me. I didn't have to act like I might be dead in a year. I might be, but why live in a dirty apartment until then?

"Then last summer I started getting transfusions every three weeks. At first I felt fine. I ran, went to the gym, and stopped drinking. I was basically in better physical and emotional health than I was five years earlier. So I didn't consider myself a sick per-son. If I did, then I would be sick. I considered myself a well per-son who might have occasional bouts of things going wrong with him. And I thought, that's a better attitude. Otherwise I'd fantasize the worst things happening to me.

"So I thought of it as a potentially chronic condition. But I thought of life as a chronic illness. I always knew I would be dead someday. Now there was a chance it would be sooner. Maybe not. Millions of chronic diseases exist in the world—some far worse than AIDS—that people live with. There might also be new drugs and treatments. But it was almost like a game. I liked playing games and solving puzzles, and if I approached it as a puzzle and each day learned another little piece and gradually filled in the boxes across and down, someday I'd finish the puzzle. I always did. Sometimes I wrote the wrong clue but later found the right one. That was the way my health worked too.

"But then a few months ago I became sick and caved in. I decided to take my own life rather than fight a losing battle. I knew I'd have to go back to the hospital. I had been there fifteen times in the previous five years, and never before in my entire life. It just wasn't worth it anymore. I locked my apartment door, counted up how many pills I'd need to do it, and turned off the light. I sat there in the dark for several minutes. At the last possible second I reached for the phone, called my physician, and was hospitalized."

The balance between hope and despair, between anticipation of life or death can be difficult to maintain. Roger Babson, the gay man living in an AIDS residence, reported, "I went to see *Gypsy* last week and thought, 'This could be my last Broadway show, the last big night out I have. Let me enjoy it. Next week I may become deathly ill.' I don't dote on the thought that it might be the last. I haven't given up hope that I'll live long enough to see a cure, or that other drugs will come out to make me live longer. But I'm not going to get my hopes up either. I'm cautious. I've seen so many friends die—it shows me what limited time I have. AIDS has robbed me of the life I had, of achieving high goals. I try to remain prepared to accept a short life span, and still hope for a long one. But it's difficult when I have been lying in bed, feeling miserable with a high fever. I tend to be more morbid, final: this is it. When you have AIDS and a problem arises, you can't help but think, is this *it,* the beginning of a debilitating illness after which I die, the beginning of The End? I wonder, will this be the case of pneumonia that kills me? Or will I recover and be able to go out and walk the streets and socialize? There's no answer. Only time will tell." The term *it* now has a new meaning—it's no longer sex appeal or id, as in 'she's got it.' The term now connotes death. In both cases—before and now—it refers to the unspoken.

Roger continues, "When I have pains in my stomach or fever, more philosophical understandings of my situation don't amount to a hill of beans. When I'm feeling lousy, that's all I'm concerned about. I don't expect myself to be Mr. Understanding. Friends and relatives try to inspire hope in me. I take those as kind but unrealistic gestures. I can't fool myself into hoping there's going to be something when I think there's not—not in my time."

Aaron Eliot, a nonbelieving Jew, lacks faith or an overarching rationale or sense of order underlying the epidemic. Instead he believes that HIV results from bad luck, and he becomes depressed. "I never thought of HIV as a punishment. People say, 'Oh, you're being punished or something.' No, I was just unfortunate to be in New York City when this thing took off. It was bad timing and bad luck that I was gay when nobody knew what was happening.

"After my initial diagnosis, everything seemed to go into a remission. But that's the luck of the cards too. I could get meningitis or CMV [cytomegalovirus, an opportunistic infection in AIDS] or pneumonia and go quickly. My doctor's probably amazed that I'm still around after three and a half years. I attribute it to chance. I was in very good shape and had the luck of the wheel. The lucky can perhaps last a few years. I had also always been a health nut." Yet he still feels a need to find a larger explanation. His depression may cause or result from his belief in luck; the two phenomena appear to be closely intertwined. Although not as pernicious as belief in a punishing God, luck too closely follows and feeds feelings of depression.

Fatalism and hopelessness often accompany depression without HIV. Aaron, unable to leave his apartment more than once every few days because of AIDS-related fatigue, explains, "HIV is a very lonely disease. Friends tell me to move upstate, but that scares me to death. I'm scared to stay where I am but scared to go. What would I be going for? I'm going to die in two years anyway. I wonder should I do this or that. What am I planning this or that for? Why make this phone call? My life is at a standstill, in limbo, hell."

Arlene Chambers also experiences this stoppage of her life. "I always wanted to be happy before I died—be with somebody for once, have somebody care about me. Life's passing me by, and I'm just standing still. When I found out, everything was thrown out the window. Everything's still on hold." She too returned to drugs, perhaps because of such feelings. Stasis scares her as an intimation of eventual death, a sense, she feels, of annihilation that awaits. This sense of limbo, and what it represents, urges her on but overwhelms her too.

This anticipation of death can also disturb friends and family. Olana Ramirez no longer uses drugs but frequently becomes depressed. She does not minimize, though her husband does and she is tempted to. "I'm tired all the time and short of breath. Everybody tells me it's because I'm heavy. But I was heavy before and didn't feel this. Sometimes I talk and forget what I'm saying. That scares me. I think, 'God, am I going crazy?' Suppose I go outside one day and forget where I live? Things like that come to my mind and my husband looks at me and says, 'You think of the dumbest things.' But I say, 'No. Look what's happening to me. I forget things. One day I could just go blank!' I shouldn't think about that but I do. What difference does it make if it's today or tomorrow? I stay indoors a lot. I also dream very seldom. When I do it's terrible, vicious, mean. Why can't I dream something nice?"

So-called major depression—clearly justifying psychiatric treatment with medications—arises as well. But this condition appeared only in those who had previous histories of major psychiatric disorders, such as major depression or substance abuse. Infected individuals more often experience milder "situational" depression.

Anxiety emerged in conjunction with fear of possible symptoms and their medical and social implications. Wilma Smith worried about "every little pimple." Maurice Bradford said, "I fear most no one being there if I become ill."

HIV separates prior, current, and future views of the self. To keep the self intact, the illness triggers a "will to wholeness." Minimization is one way to bridge the gap between past and present, reducing this tension. Alfie Montoya, for example, clung to the belief that he was "okay except for this bug inside me." But other individuals employed different strategies. Wilma succeeded by acknowledging that change had occurred, now thinking of herself as "HIV Wilma." Roy Gifford, who studied biology, conceptualized part of himself as continuing on, untouched by the virus, after his death. Kerry Musgrove eventually saw himself as completely diseased and fell into despair. Individuals incorporated changes from the illness into their lives differently, and altered these approaches over time.

These men and women put together narratives of their lives that made sense for them. Those who felt an irreconcilable rupture between their past and present selves usually experienced depression as well. Maurice Bradford, the health care administrator, in many ways became a different person, seen differently by himself and others. "I continue to be amazed that the things I read happening to people with this illness are happening to me. I'm not prepared for it. I've never been prepared for bad things happening to me. I admit I've been called 'Naive Nell from the Country,' but this has all just been too much." For him, a broken identity and a sense of depression occurred simultaneously.

In conjunction with such psychological distress, Raoul and others frequently ponder suicide. As Ken Landers said, "I hear about and see other people living with outward signs of Kaposi's, but I don't know how I could deal with that. I struggle already as it is. I saw a young man with lesions all over his face. I've always been very sensitive about the way I look and get very neurotic about any blemishes. If KS came like that, I might take a pill and say goodbye." Suicidal thoughts can thus result in part from medical symptoms that threaten one's self, particularly if it is fragile to begin with.

Suicidal thoughts shape experiences of the illness itself, offering the possibility of escape if the illness worsens. "I'm determined to keep living," Roy said, "until such time as living doesn't appeal, though I don't know when that would be." Yet like a horizon that seems ever to recede as one approaches it, and which is thus never reached, suicide remains a foreseeable but unattained point. Many individuals adapt to stages they thought would be wholly unacceptable. Patients then feel they would take their lives if they reached a still more advanced stage, but find when they arrive at it that they are able to cope with it too. They then put off even further the stage at which they imagine they would kill themselves. Several studies have suggested that people with HIV have an increased rate of suicide, though later studies have indicated otherwise. Nonetheless many individuals recurringly consider suicide as an option. It provides, if nothing else, a sense of freedom, choice, and control over their deaths. If one cannot determine whether one dies or what happens afterward, one can still decide when and how to bring closure. One doesn't have to lose mental and bodily functions while continuing to "live" through artificial life supports.

Contemplating dependency on others and the accompanying humiliation also triggers suicidal thoughts. As Arthur Williams put it, "I prefer to believe that since my T-cell count is high, I won't get AIDS. If I do, I'd probably kill myself. Definitely. I'd take a drug overdose. If I couldn't get cyanide tablets, I would kill myself some other way. I wouldn't want to go through it, or put anyone else through it, having to take care of me. I don't know who I could get to take care of me when I have diarrhea in bed and need someone to clean it up. I would rather kill myself. Being sick is the least of it—it's just no way to live. A couple of weeks is one thing, but with something incurable like AIDS I wouldn't want to live. I don't have the cyanide pills lined up, and I might change my mind. I don't even think I'll get AIDS. But I don't like to talk about it either."

HIV-land generally does not support suicidal thoughts, though they are common. George Sullivan said, "A friend, white as a sheet and thin as a toothpick, called me up on a snowy night and said he would give me $1,000 to get a gun and shoot him. He was in a lot of pain. But I wasn't about to murder somebody, no matter what."

In response to such feelings of depression and stasis, HIV impels a search for movement. Aaron Eliot and others, when asked what they look forward to, immediately said "traveling"—going to places they have never been, to expand horizons that seem to be shrinking. These patients feel stuck and seek at least temporary escape. Aaron elaborated, "I'd love to go to parts of the United States I've never seen and do things I haven't done: take a train across Canada to Alaska, then down the Pacific Northwest and back across the country. But I know I never will. I'll try to make do with a trip on the Staten Island ferry." Unfortunately it wasn't clear he'd even be able to do that.

Yet HIV revitalizes many, impelling them to preserve a sense of themselves as alive. "I try to be optimistic," Olana said. "I know that if I don't fight, I will die. Sadly, it took me getting HIV to learn what it means to live."

Those with substance abuse, in particular, now restructure their sense of time. As Gloria Higgens said, "I have had to deal with this illness step by step, something I'm not used to doing."

Many adopt a tone of resurrection and rebirth. Twelve-step programs often provide models that help with HIV. As Gerry Galvez, who had made "a pact with God," said, "I consistently ask the Lord to give me the strength to deal with this virus. I feel I've been given a reprieve"—as if it was divinely ordained. "Most of my life I've been a loner, and I've come back into the world as a valuable and productive human being." She has recreated herself, embodying elements of symbolic immortality that were absent before. A new social and moral self has emerged.

Transcendence over death and the relief of stigma can be achieved in certain basic ways. People vary and fluctuate as crises come and go. Yet through time and the course of these lives, essential patterns persist. In their absence, despair and anxiety more likely occur, along with fatalism, hopelessness, and feelings of stasis. Those who are unable to remake their sense of self and their world have difficulty integrating their lives before and after infection. Suicidal thoughts arise in conjunction with these problems and as a result of HIV stresses, including humiliation and rage over anticipated dependency on others. Yet this distress can also prompt a search for movement, growth, and redefinitions of the self. Such creative change can be facilitated through several of the patterns of adaptation described, including engagement in HIV-land, volunteerism, spirituality, and connectedness to family. Through these means HIV can revitalize the self, reconfiguring the individual on many levels. The illness thus becomes recast—it is about not only stigma and loss but recreation and rebirth.

ELEVEN

The Odds: *Risky Behavior*

THE RANGE OF ADAPTATIONS to HIV also has important implications for health behavior. A patient's response to the illness can affect his own and others' health for good or bad. These patterns thus offer critical lessons in disease prevention.

Of Flesh and Dreams

Sexual acts with another person can provide a sense of freedom, even if briefly, from feelings of rejection, stasis, and death. Yet unless safe sex is practiced, dangers lurk—the risk of infecting partners or reinfecting oneself. Thus individuals face a tension between desire and potential danger—escaping from or potentially causing death.

Some individuals continue the same level of unsafe sexual activity, or practice more. Todd Crenshaw, who had bemoaned the loss of his socioeconomic status, said, "I've been known to lapse in practicing safe sex. It's always mutual. The person on top is positive or at least knows I am. I prefer that they're positive—so my lapse depends on my partner's health status. If he's negative and wants me to engage in risky behavior, I'll always use a condom. But I feel that as I've already been infected, what's the difference if I get infected again? Thus far I've been lucky—I've just had PCP and candida and fatigue. It doesn't matter to me that I may get reinfected, because I'm not very happy with the quality of my life anyway, the way it's turned out. Before I got sick I was in the process of buying a coop. Now I'm on DAS [New York City disability benefits], which is like welfare. I'm not working and have to associate with junkies. I feel like a failure—I no longer have the dream of success in America. I have not lived up to what I should have. Yet if not for DAS, I'd be living on the street. To afford food I have to pay my rent late.

"When I lost control over my health, I lost control over my life. I exorcize that through self-destructive behavior, hurting myself through unsafe sex, abusing my body. I've probably reinfected myself many times. But I have no control over other aspects of my life. I'm getting back at doctors who don't take me seriously unless I have a five-hundred-degree temperature. If I get infected with a different type of virus, maybe I'll develop other infections: toxoplasmosis. Many times I find myself picking up things I'm not attracted to because it's nice to know that at least somebody wants me even though I have AIDS.

"I also escape by not taking my medicine. It's another form of self-destructive behavior. Taking medicine reminds me that things aren't going the way they should, that I'm sick and have AIDS—which equals death. I might lose my sight or develop meningitis. I'm tired of waking up in the morning, brushing my teeth, opening the medicine cabinet and seeing all these pills, reminding me that I'm positive, that this disease is terminal and that I'm not in control. Every three or four months I stop taking them all, because what's the use? I've been on AZT for over two years, and studies say that it only works for about a year or year and a half anyway.

So it's not doing me any good. Yet if I don't take these pills, I may get thrush or something else. There's just no break. I push and push and push and can't get away from it.

"I no longer trust doctors now either. A few years ago one hospital practically killed me because a medical resident decided to discharge me too early. Goddam residents and interns see me and don't know my history or what the hell's going on. I have to give them the entire story, and they don't care. I was almost a physicians' assistant before I got sick, and I know as much about the disease as they do."

For Tony Wilmot, a thirty-five-year-old Italian-American gay man, "Sex is the only way I can get real skin-to-skin contact, get close to people, have somebody kiss me or love me. I'm willing to do anything, including unsafe sex, to get that. Usually I'm already drunk.

"Eighty percent of the time I practice safer sex," he explains. "But recently, for example, a guy and I rented a room and didn't have a condom. We were already hot to trot. We were more scared about the place than about having sex. It was more dangerous—a sleazebag hotel, forty dollars for a single bed. I've never been to a dive before. I had to blank it out and pretend I was somewhere else. It's hard for me to change my 'social-sexual' life"—the term reveals the confluence of the two. Sex defines his social life, and his social life revolves around sex.

"I really don't care so much about myself as about other people. I didn't care whether he fucked me and came in my ass—it felt great—or if I gave him a blow job and he came in my mouth. I don't care whether we do unsafe sex. I take pleasure in being fucked without a condom. But I let them do it on the condition they don't ejaculate inside me"—though this provision is clearly precarious.

His riskiness stems partly from his background. "I'm a foster kid, adopted. My parents tried to abort me even before I was born. Whenever I travel to another part of the country, I look in the phone book for someone with my last name. To be foster is to be cut off from people who couldn't care less. It's a loss of identity. Nobody claims me as their own. At Christmas I wrote a letter to every one of my siblings, as well as to my foster parents and my real parents. The only person I got a response from was my real mother.

"My foster parents had twenty-five children by the time I graduated from college. The state named them the Foster Parents of the Year. But we kids didn't think so. My foster mother was herself a foster child. We were deprived of any emotional or close skin-to-skin contact."

Unfortunately Tony's practice of unsafe sex, though traceable to his background, is far from unique. Many look for reasons to believe their partner is HIV negative. Kerry Musgrove said, "I went out one evening with a nurse and at the end of the night he said, 'Do you want to come to my house?' and I said, 'Well, okay,' and it ended up he wanted to have sex. I said, 'You do?' And he said, 'Yes.' I said, 'Well, aren't you afraid?' And he said, 'Well, no. Why? As long as you don't do anything that makes me catch it from you.' We actually had a nice time, and I learned something from it. For a long time I viewed myself as unattractive, unappealing, and untouchable—unlikely to have any kind of relationship, either short- or long-term. I don't feel that way anymore. I don't have a lover, but that doesn't mean I can't or that I have to view myself as unsexual, unable to have sex ever again."

Unfortunately such feelings of low self-worth can foster unsafe sex. Kerry continues, "The summer after I started volunteering at GMHC, I met Jack, a very sweet doctor from the South. I went home with him and he asked, 'Do you want me to use a condom?' I remember thinking, 'Well, he's a doctor, so he must be okay.' I'll never forget that. We didn't have a very long or even a very sexual relationship, but he did fuck me a few times in July and August of '84. Well, he died two and a half years ago, right before I found out I had AIDS."

"Even after a year of working as an AIDS volunteer and understanding all about the disease, I still let somebody fuck me!"

Aaron Eliot similarly explained, "I was seeing, on a steady basis, an ultraconservative guy who was a professor. I didn't go with anybody else. I saw him until I got sick, when he came over and wanted to talk to me. I said, 'Maybe you should be tested yourself.' And then he told me about a friend of his whom he had seen and who had died of KS in '83. He had never told me this before. I thought he was monogamous and that I was perfectly safe. We practiced unsafe sex and I thought, 'Here's a guy who never goes out, doesn't go to bars or cruise, whom I had met many, many years ago.' Now he's sick himself."

Unsafe sex occurs because of fatalism too. Roy Gifford, for example, said, "When I tested positive I was also newly out. I felt, 'Gee, I should have been the biggest whore in Manhattan. Being careful didn't really matter.' I would have liked to have been a little more adventurous, but I was gun shy. Yet the end result wound up the same. I might as well have enjoyed life more. At least I would have had memories of wonderful times instead of feelings of limitation."

The virus may be further transmitted because of uncertainty about what is, in fact, safe. Maurice Bradford had "practiced 'modified' safe sex: things not as safe as they could be—such as oral sex without protection. I wouldn't do that now. As you learn more, there's not much that's safe. But my lover rejected me, then came back and wanted sex but without protection, which I thought was strange." For various reasons, HIV-positive individuals thus place themselves at risk for being reinfected with other strains of the virus. In the case of other viruses, it is known that different strains—some more virulent than others, the degree of exposure, and the route of transmission can all affect the course of illness. Unsafe sex can also spread other diseases.

HIV-infected individuals decide about their degree of vulnerability. Leonard Barber said he was "not afraid of reinfection. The jury is still out on how self-destructive that is. I've agreed to unprotected anal sex with a friend who is also HIV positive. I don't really think his strain of virus is that much more virulent than mine, otherwise he'd be in worse shape than he is. His T-cells are okay, and he's been positive as long as I have. Of course, I'm not a doctor." Yet he and other patients nonetheless make such medical diagnoses and determinations. He adds, "Not being concerned about getting infected is a great liberation. I don't have to be afraid of getting it—which profoundly distorts the lives of HIV negatives. I know young people who've come out since HIV who feel too inhibited to enjoy sex without a condom." The infected gay men with whom I spoke thus risked reexposing themselves more than exposing others, specifically being the receptive partner in unprotected anal intercourse with a partner of unknown or negative HIV status. These men may nonetheless be exposing their partners to the virus.

Unsafe sex also occurs among those who rely heavily on religion, which can relieve responsibility but lead to passivity. Jason Gillian is highly religious and feels his illness is in God's hands. Yet at one point he had unsafe sex as a receptive partner. "I missed Ben and wanted to feel another man inside me," he explained. Jason risked both reinfection and the possibility of exposing the other man to the virus. In believing that God will protect him, Jason fears reinfection less than others.

Minimization can also predispose toward risky sexual activity. Those who feel, in effect, that nothing's wrong with them face less of a barrier in engaging in potentially dangerous behavior. Todd Crenshaw, too, frustrated and depressed over his lost dreams, lets his sexual partner's potential pleasure outweigh his own avoidance of reinfection.

Many engage in riskier sexual activities because of altered judgment resulting from drugs. The conflict between knowing a behavior is dangerous and wanting to engage in it anyway can be difficult to reconcile. Elsa Diaz said about herself, "There was a day girl and a night girl"—one used drugs, the other didn't. As Arlene Chambers said, "My boyfriend and I don't discuss HIV at all. Just 'How do you feel?' 'I'm fine, how do you feel?' 'Fine.' That's it. We don't dwell on it, because whenever we talk about it we get upset. We're living another day and that's it. We practice safe sex but not all the time. He says it's uncomfortable, and it irritates me, so we rarely use it." She and her boyfriend also continue to use drugs, further erasing the potential conflict.

Failure to practice safer sex can result from other interpersonal problems. As Gerry Galvez said, "For a while I didn't push safe sex with my husband, so we'd get along better. I couldn't convince him."

Formal and informal discussion in HIV-land encourages prevention and safer sexual practices. Yet private resistance to safer sex continues.

HIV-land, cohesive in some ways but weak in others, arises in part from gay culture, which differs from other cultures in that younger members are not raised in it from birth but enter it by choice later in life. Still, older gay men often feel responsible for instructing younger counterparts. As Roy Gifford said, "A straight couple asked me to talk to their son who was just coming out. My opening statement to him was, 'Here is a bag of rubbers. Use them or don't worry about *the virus* getting you, because *I* will.' "

Some members of HIV-land hold very realistic views of the illness, which nonetheless lead to unsafe sex. Matt Winchell, for example, has "no illusions about my prognosis. I expect I will die in two years. Why bother with condoms if I'm only risking getting reinfected?" Yet even as the passive partner in anal intercourse, he could potentially infect the other person, though the risk is lower. "Slipups" of unsafe sex, increasingly discussed in the media, have further legitimized discussion of such events.

Many reduce their high-risk sexual behavior. George Sullivan said, "I have been promiscuous, but a lot of that was pre-AIDS, and of course I'm a different age and settled down now. AIDS has also incredibly affected the gay community's policies, though a lot of people out there are still just playing Russian roulette." As he indicates, people develop policies they may not always follow. "Before, I would go into the park at night, looking for anonymous sex. A few times since, I've still been unsafe with one person. That relationship started before I accepted the fact I was positive, and I couldn't find a way of beginning to wear a condom after not having worn one for so long. I'm still in touch with him and see him socially, but it's not been sexual. When I was involved in unsafe sex, I wondered, 'Why am I doing this?' I felt guilt and then corrected the situation by just not having sex for a while."

Others abstain altogether. Jenny Singer said, "When I first found out I had the virus, my whole desire for sex dropped off. I couldn't care less if I ever had sex again. Then it became very hard for me to get into having sex again, especially safe sex. What if I infected or contaminated somebody by having sex with them? That changed everything. To have oral sex I have to put a piece of Saran wrap over my genitalia. I feel I'm a germ, not sexy. I also don't want to touch anyone else directly because I could get something from them."

Donny Sotelo, who described himself as a "garbage head," now abstains because he feels no relationship would have a future. "I used condoms once in my life and didn't like them, so I've had no sex at all in the past three years. If the woman initiated the thing about having safe sex, it might be a good relationship. But as far as I'm concerned, there's no future with me and a female for sex—that's it, that's as far as we can go. So there's no future for an HIV-positive person in a relationship because there's a limitation on what they can do. You can't have unprotected sex. What if she wanted to get married or deeply involved? I wouldn't want to hurt her or start something I couldn't finish. So I shy away. To get married or involved with somebody is condemning her to live with somebody who's gonna die—knowing he's gonna die. I wouldn't want that on nobody. If you care for somebody, you don't do that." Such abstention can be difficult for many others.

Whether HIV status is disclosed also affects the likelihood that safer sex will be practiced. Matt said, "I could have infected a lot of guys if I had wanted to. Many will let me fuck them or will fuck me without a rubber. It's amazing. Status is not discussed. Like meeting somebody in a dirty bookstore and then having sex there. They're begging me to fuck them, or trying to fuck me without a rubber. This happens not infrequently. And I'm surprised by that. When there is communication involved and people are talking, it's only brought up about a third to half of the time.

"If I go to a bookstore to have sex, nobody there is asking people their status. I'm not going to come in their mouths. But I'm not going to tell them I'm positive. They've made the decision that they feel okay with that, so if they want to suck me, fine. There have been times when guys in situations like that—pickups—have gotten me going enough that they have gotten inside me without a rubber, not knowing I'm positive. I feel bad and guilty about that. It's happened a few times in the passion of sex.

"But they're having sex they are comfortable having with anybody. My status is obviously not an issue with them because they're not asking me. So they're having what they consider safe sex. Everybody is safe in their own mind. Is oral sex safe? Is sodomy without any coming safe? I think it is. And they obviously think it is too, because they do it. Some people would say, 'I could never do that with somebody who's positive if I'm negative.' And frankly, if I were negative, I probably wouldn't do it either. But it could be just a psychological barrier. Scientifically I believe it's safe." Still, he would be uncomfortable if he were not already infected. In short, a double standard often operates. Bedroom ethics remain murky—an oxymoron—and people do what they can "get away with." He and others practice an implicit policy of *caveat emptor*. In part, he and others take this approach because the passion and excitement of sex is a release for them, a chance to escape death and constraint while experiencing an all-encompassing union with another human being.

"I don't feel an obligation to disclose that I'm positive," he continued, "but I do feel an obligation not to expose people. I feel absolutely no possibility of transmission exists in oral sex when their dick is in my mouth. A year and a half ago I felt that there wasn't a risk to a negative person fucking me with Nonoxynol-9 [an antiviral included in many lubricants]. So I did that a couple of times with someone. I feel I'm not really good enough to fuck other guys. So a hot guy coming inside me excites me sexually. I'm getting a charge from somebody better than me. I wouldn't let anybody do that now unless they really argued for it. I've changed my mind." Thus Matt fears not reinfection but infecting someone else. As he also indicates, sexual activities vary depending on whether the partner is anonymous (e.g., a "one-night stand" or "pickup") or better known.

Needle sharing also spreads the virus. As noted earlier, those who continue to inject drugs often see meager impediments to using each other's injection apparatus.

Potions and Poisons

Adherence to medical regimens depends upon how individuals respond to the disease. Many see medications as potentially toxic, of limited benefit, inconvenient, and as harbingers of illness and death. Lorraina Ortiz said, "I hate clocking myself and getting up at four in the morning to take AZT. I don't think: this is AZT for the virus. I don't think what's it's for. I just take it like aspirin or, in the past, valium."

Yet the controversy surrounding AZT lessens compliance. Some delay starting it. Many who believe HIV represents a government experiment also avoid medications.

Substance abuse precipitates poor compliance and misconceptions about treatment. Dede Alwin said, "I don't like putting something toxic inside my body. What if I have to detox from it later?"—even though these drugs are medical, not recreational. She also blames AZT for her T-cells dropping after she started it. "And I get tired of taking pills, of the frequency of the doses. I have to keep an eye on my watch to make sure I take AZT four times a day, and I have my other medicines spaced out too. I keep one eye on my watch, hour after hour, day after day. It gets boring. It's work, and I sometimes forget. So much of these drugs goes in me constantly that I've thought, 'What harm would there be if I miss a dose?' The timer beeps and I take the pill and throw the timer to the side. When it beeps again my son or my husband runs over with it. It beeps at five o'clock in the morning. A few times I've opened the pillbox at night and can't remember if I took the pill or not. I know I woke up and stopped the stupid sound from going off, but I forget if I swallowed a pill or just turned off the sound. I hate having to carry that damn thing all over the place. Sometimes I purposely forget. Two or three times a month I go off my regular routine. I start thinking, 'What if this toxic drug does something irreversible?' I'm pretty healthy, but who's to say? I could build tolerance to the full dosage, and then if I need AZT in the future there'll be nothing because I'd already built a tolerance to it." Misconceptions arise, modeled on drugs of abuse. Resistance may develop to antibiotics, but "tolerance" develops only with the use of addictive substances.

Dede continues, "My concept over the years of taking medication has been to get well. But this is not going to happen now. Despite all this medicine, I can still get sick. So my old concept of taking medicine to get better doesn't work." She and others implicitly make a risk-benefit calculation, and the concept of prevention compels little. Yet "if my doctor asks, I tell him I'm still taking it, even though I'm not."

As a result of drug use, Gary Stevens, who thought HIV was "just a blood disorder," refuses to follow his medical regimens. "I was taking INH [Isoniazid] for a touch of TB exposure, but I stopped. I didn't have a cough or tiredness or symptoms. I didn't tell the doctor I was stopping. Some things you keep to yourself and don't tell the world. I just stopped on my own because I started doing drugs. Once I do illegal drugs, I don't take no other drugs. I don't like to put a drug on top of a drug. We HIV carriers have the virus, but it's limited. It doesn't overact. But if I take drugs on top of AZT, I would explode because everything in my body would erupt. Like combustion. I think a person can do without AZT. You have to deal with health naturally. Although I use heroin as a chemical, my body doesn't react as much as if I used AZT too. AZT without drugs made me nervous; my whole body felt like it was going to erupt inside like a volcano. That's how people die—by taking two sedatives together.

"I also don't know whether medicine will help me because if I stop it, it will make the virus come on full force. If I take it, I have to take it the rest of my life, right? And what if I decide I don't want to anymore. It'll kill me faster." He sees the possibility of withdrawal as if AZT were an addictive drug.

Gary defends his attitude by viewing HIV as fated. "Whatever happens will happen anyway because the Lord let it be. We all got a destiny, a number. Whatever has been said and done to me has been said and done. If this is a judgment put upon me, I just have to deal with that. It's not like I'm the baddest person in the world."

Other misconceptions about HIV prompt poor adherence to medication regimens. Many drug users asked questions that reveal confusion about the illness and its progression. "Does all HIV turn to AIDS?" Reynaldo Fernandez, who felt his "seed" was "poison," asked. His uncertainty reflects that of researchers as the epidemic enters its second decade, with many infected individuals still developing few if any symptoms. Yet he also asked, "Did everyone with AIDS have HIV first?" suggesting his wider uncertainty about these two terms. The progression from infection to death remains frightening but has not always occurred.

Some drug users, however, are more amenable to medication. "I put poison in my body anyway," Olana Ramirez said. "So I go along with AZT." As she has already risked much, her body is now less inviolate to her.

Gay men as well as drug users experience difficulty taking medications. Roy Gifford says, "I allow myself each month one drug-free day, a day for just being normal, leaving my pillbox at home and not hearing the beeper go off every few hours. Otherwise my life is blocked off in four-hour increments, which makes me very aware of time passing. Also, if I'm out for dinner and my beeper goes off, I feel everybody is thinking, 'What's that?' I always have to think, 'Gee what time is it? Will I be in transit when I have to take my pill?' At first I was very concerned about taking everything on schedule. HIV ruled my life. Then I decided it was ludicrous and I was taking it all much too seriously. So I allowed myself the luxury of forgetting about it. Now, once a week, if it's inconvenient to take a pill, I just don't bother. I say, 'It's in the wind, the hell with it.' My drug-free days once a month or 'as needed' give me some sense of freedom and normality. That's my way of dealing with it: my reward. I allow myself one period to act out, not any set time." Of note, he developed PCP immediately after one such week, but he doesn't trace this event to reduced medication. He seeks freedom from medications that remind him that time is "passing" and limited, and that he is not "normal."

Responses to rejection and threats of annihilation have high stakes. Feelings about the self can hamper health inadvertently or unconsciously. Low self-esteem, exacerbated by HIV, as well as a sense of fatalism about the illness, can foster unsafe sex. Drug use, minimization of the illness, and a belief that fate is "all in God's hands" can also lower impediments to risky behavior. Other individuals abstain from sexual encounters altogether as a result of the illness.

Adherence to medication varies too, based on beliefs about and stances toward the disease. Thus responses to the illness strongly shape approaches to risk.

TWELVE

The Second Closet:
Disclosures

BECAUSE OF STIGMA, infected men and women face difficult decisions about disclosing their status—determining who, when, and what to tell. HIV status can precipitate other difficult revelations, sometimes necessitating a double coming out—as, for example, both infected and gay. Adaptations to the illness affect these decisions, which in turn can lead to situations in which the virus may more readily be transmitted.

Disclosure of HIV infection differs in some ways from other types of disclosure, including that of homosexuality. As Tony Wilmot said, "Telling friends I'm HIV positive is not the same as telling them I'm gay. I don't know how to escape, laugh it off, or say to people, 'Yeah, I'm HIV positive,' like I do when I say I'm gay. People react differently, no matter how close or distant they are. They give me a big hug, or say, 'I'm sorry,' which they've never said before when I told them something traumatic. Or they don't know how to react. The types of information are different"—that is, one means possible death (despite the advent of new, improved medications), the other doesn't.

Tony continues, "I'm afraid to get close to anybody or go to a bar and pick someone up and go home with them, because as soon as I tell them I'm HIV positive, I won't even be able to make it out the front door. I thought being gay was bad enough."

Disclosure of HIV status can lead to more complete and painful rejection. As Matt Winchell described, "Some guys can't handle that I'm positive when I tell them. The worst experience was with a guy I dated last summer. We met over the phone-sex lines, spoke for a month beforehand, and got along great. We finally got together and had two dates. He was nuts about me. On the third date I told him I was positive. We had a few more dates and then he broke it off, citing all these reasons: that I was too critical and negative. We had these long discussions about my problems. Being rejected hurt me a lot. It took me a year to figure out that he was crazy about me till he knew I was positive. He had not been tested. I was furious with him that he used this subterfuge and was afraid to admit it. For months I was pissed off at him and screamed at him in my head. I'm good enough even though I'm positive. We could still have had good sex. I have to understand it's irrational and people are allowed to have those fears because this is scary. AIDS and HIV are illogical. Plague is illogical. I can't expect people to do what is logical. But I got angry at this guy's dishonesty. He was too cowardly to come out and say, 'It scares the hell out of me that you're positive.' He was too fucking wimpy to get tested, and then he got mad at me because I had been, even though I'm asymptomatic and totally healthy.

"That's why for a long time my standard thing to say was that I hadn't been tested but was probably positive because I had had sex with guys who were positive. I wouldn't come right out and say it, because back then hardly anybody was tested. So my ex-boyfriend to this day doesn't know I'm positive; we broke up before I was ready to tell him. But I did plant a very strong seed in his mind that I probably was positive, even, '98 percent probable

HIV.' " Clearly the label itself carries a unique weight. Of note, Matt does not feel guilty that he partially lied, because he communicated a message of sex being potentially risky—of *caveat emptor.*

Some people don't even tell about themselves when others disclose to them. Gary Stevens said, "One friend put her confidence in me that she's HIV positive. But I never told her about myself. She might be the one I have sex with someday. People are also very slick. That's the way I was. So I don't trust anybody. I trust only a few people now—really only one person, my mother. I don't trust my brother. A wall is there, a block as far as letting people get on the good side of me or close to me. That's why I haven't told anybody.

"I like spending time with people who are HIV positive, especially if they don't know I'm HIV. It's better for them because they think I'm straight—that is, HIV negative—and am still spending time with them. That makes me feel good. It's reverse psychology."

More complete lies can also result. "I tested positive in prison," Arlene Chambers, the African-American woman who didn't like support groups, told me. "The first thing I thought was, 'Oh my God, everybody's going to know. I'm not going to tell anybody because they'll look at me differently.' I like to be accepted. So getting hit with that, I thought, 'Wow! Nobody's going to want to be bothered with me, especially when the population in the prison finds out.' I wanted to die, to kill myself. I lied about it like everybody else, and said they didn't know what they were talking about. No one came to me and said, 'I identify with you.' There was just a hush-hush like everybody was pointing their finger at me and thinking 'She has it!' Later on I found out I wasn't the only one there who had it, and I was angry because one person who pointed her finger at me had HIV too and was trying to take the focus off herself and put it on me.

"Later, on the AZT, my skin and nails started getting darker, which bothered me. So I started polishing my fingernails burgundy red. I never used to do that unless I was going out to dinner. My skin color also got dark. I started lying and telling people I had been in California and that the sun did this to me.

"My cousin has a law degree from Harvard, but I still can't come out and tell her I have the virus. It might frighten her so she might think, 'I'd better not use that glass,' even though she may have read thousands and thousands of papers about the disease. To come face to face with somebody that has it is different. She might not think that, but I'm scared to take the chance.

"My daughter lives with me now but still doesn't know I have the virus. Even though my mother and I are close, I just can't tell her either. I would like to but can't bring myself to do it. If I tell her she would be very overprotective. 'You'd better get your rest, you'd better eat, you shouldn't party.' She'd watch to make sure I didn't buy beer. People have a lot of things wrong with them that they don't broadcast. I'm also afraid of telling my family I'm HIV because we just buried my sister who died of full-blown AIDS. It makes it harder. I'm afraid they'll disown me. My sister and brother don't tell me all their business. I know that for a fact. So I don't tell them." Secrecy breeds secrecy.

Yet her concealment is all the more surprising, given that her husband had kept his positive HIV status from her and infected her. "He didn't tell me he was sick and made me think everything was okay. I didn't find out until he went into the hospital and the doctors told me. He said he was going to the doctor for a urine infection. He was hospitalized, and the doctor told me I should get myself tested. I waited six months because I was scared." The fear of rejection is so strong that despite having been lied to, Arlene was not honest but lied to others.

HIV status nonetheless becomes the stuff of rumors. "Although I didn't talk to nobody about it for two years, someone saw me and went back to New Jersey and started telling people I was dying from AIDS. I didn't even tell this person. But my face used to be a little rounder and had sunk in. The rumor hit quickly."

Her secrecy has other costs as well. "The hardest part about HIV now is not being able to make it a normal part of my life where I can talk to somebody and say, 'Well, I'm going to see the doctor tomorrow,' or 'I have to take Pentamidine,' or 'Damn, I feel tired,' and tell people straight out what's going on. I don't like hiding it. It makes me lonely." To manage this secrecy takes energy and concentration, and increases one's sense of isolation.

Yvette Bing also doesn't disclose, though she too had not been told. "The only ones that know are my counselor in my drug program and the lady that did the testing. Although my husband and me ain't together, was I gonna tell him I'm HIV positive? He was living in the street—living wherever he was living. He got in touch with me and made me feel sorry for him, so I let him come back home. But we got in a fight, and he told me then he was HIV positive. He'd be irresponsible, getting high and leaving the needle around. I'd tell him, 'Don't leave this here, somebody could come in.' But he didn't care. Then he told me he tested positive for HIV when he was in prison in 1987. He told it in a vindictive, nasty way: if he got it, then I got it too, so now I can have sex with him. That's why he told me. I don't know why he didn't say anything until now. But he was hoping I'd get it. He can be evil. If we had been getting along, I probably would have been able to tell him I was positive too. But he was too bossy.

"One day he got mad and said he got HIV from me! I called him a bastard, and he grabbed me and hit me.

"So I've told no one since. I haven't told my girlfriend. She's my lover, but I still wouldn't tell her. I tried to. But she's so bitchy. When she fights she punches me. I don't like to fight. I'm not about violence. I don't like to live like that. I'm afraid of her mouth and her fighting. My mother, when she was in the hospital before she died, said, 'That woman is gonna cause you trouble.' Maybe my mother saw something I didn't see. My mother was a wise woman. If I tell my girlfriend, she'll call me names: idiot. But I'm no idiot. She'll hit me. She gets upset and goes off and pops me in the eye. No way can I tell her."

Because of difficulties that may result from disclosures, telling often occurs in code. Maurice Bradford said, "I've not been completely honest to my lover about my situation, but I've tried to let him know. I never volunteer it because I'm afraid of being abandoned and alone. I discussed with him my problem with fluctuating T-cells, but I don't think he's put two and two together. With other people I can talk about dropping T-cell counts and they know I must be positive. He and I talk about HIV generally, but he's never come out and asked me directly if I was HIV positive. That might be his own denial. Maybe he has selective hearing and doesn't want to hear it.

"My mother does not know, either, that I'm positive, but she's concerned about my health. She asked me if I was 'all right,' meaning clean of AIDS. I told her yes, I was all right. But I still wouldn't tell her I'm positive." Both questions and answers about HIV are delivered in code that may or may not be correctly interpreted.

Even without HIV, code and innuendo play important roles in sexual encounters, both gay and straight. As Maurice explained, "With one friend I have an unspoken signal. If he wants to get laid when he's in my house, he wanders upstairs to use the bathroom on the second floor rather than the one on the first floor. He expects me to come upstairs, and we wind up having sex. We each know that."

Others besides sexual partners use codes and partial truths as well. Jill says, "They said my nephew had TB, but I think it was AIDS. He went too fast. I told people he died of TB. His other grandmother had a piece of glass put over the coffin—it was an open casket—to protect us because he had AIDS. In the projects people walk around and say, 'So-and-so has it.' You know how people talk. A guy who used to live in my building is in a wheelchair now. I think he's got AIDS. That's what his wife's sister says, but he tells everybody he's in a wheelchair because he got shot." Even obituaries in the *New York Times* often report only partial truths (e.g., listing "pneumonia" or "meningitis" rather than AIDS as the cause of death). Partial truths run the gamut, concealing the fact of HIV to varying degrees.

Failure to disclose becomes rationalized. Mitchell Walters, the Caucasian injecting drug user, said, "If I'm with a woman who is also on methadone and knows my past, I think to myself, 'She knows I might have HIV.' If she doesn't ask me to use a condom, I won't, given the fact that I hate them.

"When I can't make love it makes me feel bad about my manhood. I didn't want to tell my last girlfriend I was HIV. She told me she doesn't have periods and had an operation so she can't have kids. It felt so good not to use condoms. I could feel wetness and moisture. I started rationalizing in my mind: if her tubes are cut and she doesn't bleed or have periods, maybe she can't get it. I was going out with her for three or four months. I was really happy 'cause I had a girl. She was living with me, was my support and my best friend. But it was weird because she didn't know about the HIV. I told her I had cancer, and that's why I was on disability. I didn't feel bad and could still make love to her without using a condom partly because she couldn't get pregnant and loved sex, and I knew she had had sex with a lot of other dudes just like me—drug people with drug histories who have been with a lot of other people sexually. I really think she has HIV in her or has been exposed to it from me or from other people. She's got to; I know her history. She's my age too, and had the same amount of time out there. It was also easy to have this lie because I was the King of What's Happening—I had girls, money, and drugs."

Mitchell's attitudes suggest the difficulties faced by HIV prevention efforts. His "higher power," drawn from paganism, doesn't preclude behavior whose morality others might question. Higher powers differ in their moral implications.

Those who don't disclose don't experience discrimination. As Yvette Bing said when I asked if she had suffered discrimination or stigma because of HIV, "I haven't because I don't tell anyone I'm positive."

Not only telling but asking sexual partners about their HIV status can be a problem. Many believe what they're told. As Maurice said, "I thought my boyfriend practiced what he preached. I asked him if he had had any gay experiences before, and he said just one or two a long time ago. He was a Wall Street Republican type, so I thought he was basically okay. After he died I found out he had had more experiences than I thought."

Parents face difficult decisions as to what to tell their children and often provide only implicit or incomplete information. Olana said, "My seven-year-old doesn't know, except that mommy has to take medicine and that something is wrong with my stomach. I have a pill timer which beeps. He's used to it. When it sounds, he grabs it, opens it, and brings it to me. He always asks me, 'Did you eat your pill?' I think it's great that he's comfortable with it." The onus of having to tell him is thus also eased, even though he may know only that she takes medication, not that she's sick.

Many wait until they can better accept their HIV status before they discuss it with others. Wilma Smith, for example, could only begin to announce it to others outside her immediate family once she had ceased blaming others and come to accept it more fully herself. Adaptations to the virus strongly affect such acceptance. Participation in HIV-land, in particular, can help individuals understand the infection and discuss it with other people.

Some patients have argued that disclosure to sexual partners shouldn't be necessary, since everyone should be responsible for protecting themselves. In an ideal world, this approach would halt the epidemic. Unfortunately many individuals assume that their partners, if infected, would disclose or practice only safer sex. These data indicate that such assumptions are not always accurate. Until everyone stops making incorrect assumptions about what they are told, HIV transmission will continue. Disclosure will remain an important issue in trying to prevent the epidemic's spread.

Disclosure of HIV status presents problems for both the infected and the uninfected. As a result of revealing their HIV status, some patients have been shunned and have suffered broken relationships, violence, and the loss of housing and jobs. Lies, partial truths, and codes—acts of omission or commission—are a way around this disclosure. Rumors, true and false, spread nonetheless.

Unfortunately sexual activity—shared with all other species—is preverbal and occurs in the absence of language, or through code and innuendo. Consequently HIV often is not discussed, leading to situations in which safer sex is not practiced and the virus spreads further.

THIRTEEN

HIV and Beyond

RECENTLY A FRIEND who lives in the country by the ocean pointed out a house—a cream-colored gingerbread Victorian with white wooden doilylike trim—across the street from her. Its small front porch overlooked the bay and then the ocean beyond. In the twilight the horizon of sea seemed to stretch on forever. "A young single man bought it last year," my friend explained. "He worked on Wall Street and said he had always wanted to have a house by the sea. The neighbors all invited him over and found him very nice. A few months ago though, he suddenly died of AIDS. We all thought, 'What a shame. He finally saved up enough money to buy the house, and then he had to die."

But as a result of these interviews I saw this situation differently. I assume that when the young man bought the property he knew he was HIV positive and had a limited lifetime. It was sad that he died, but I sensed that before he did he had managed to do something he wanted.

The narratives in this book allow us to see life from these patients' own perspectives, not simply from our own. The stories proved more powerful than I had anticipated, enabling us to enter these individuals' worlds. As I look back, I realize how much I learned from these men and women. In retrospect, I had started out with several assumptions—not all clear to me at the time—about psychological distress, self-change, and narratives.

I had expected far more persistent distress and depression caused by the illness, as I found in the clinic. Suicidal thoughts do continue to surface. And HIV-infected men and women face a tenuous balance between life and death in themselves and others. In addition, they face rejection, stigma, and pain from multiple sources around them. Yet these tales display courage and persistence in the face of such odds, and teach us much about resilience—how people from even disadvantaged backgrounds find strength and respond when pushed to the limits of physical and mental endurance.

Individuals come to terms with these stresses by finding meaning in the illness and in their lives. Victor Frankl, in his book *Man's Search for Meaning,* drawing on his experiences surviving Auschwitz, wrote that human beings need purpose. Frankl quotes Nietzsche: "He who has a *why* to live can bear almost any *how.*" Faced with widespread annihilation of themselves and others around them, the men and women interviewed here seek a larger significance to their lives. This study illuminates the range of approaches they use, demonstrating not only that people seek meaning but exactly how they find it.

Individuals find strength through HIV-land, spirituality, volunteerism, and family. I was surprised that traditional values such as religion and family prove as crucial as they do. Yet patients follow these broad patterns in individual ways, shaped by personal background and experience. Survival itself becomes a creative endeavor as men and women grapple to find answers that work.

Through these broad patterns they are able to integrate illness and mortality into their lives, accepting death not just intellectually but experientially, and preparing to deal with it when it arrives. They struggle to surrender myths—even if unconscious—of immortality, and to find something to live for. I had not imagined the depths of anguish nor the heights of wisdom and insight they achieve—the troubles they had encountered in their lives but are now able to confront and discuss.

By acknowledging the possibility of death, many patients now develop an increased appreciation of the present, of the life that remains. They realize they had taken life for granted and now have stopped and changed. For me personally, they urge a message akin to Seneca's: live each day as if it were the last, and hence be prepared for, rather than frightened by, death, whenever it may arrive. These narratives thus affirm human potential and strength.

The quest for meaning extends across differences in gender, race, sexual orientation, class, and education. At first I was surprised that even those deeply embedded in the worlds of injecting drug use, who had sacrificed their lives to their addiction, still sought purpose and dignity. Much of society objectifies drug users as "other," making this group easier to ignore. Yet these stories show them as struggling people with feelings.

Spirituality proved far more important and pervasive than I had foreseen. Higher powers provide not just connectedness with a future after death, but a sense that despite rejection by other people, God is accepting and understanding. Spirituality also offers an explanation for "why me" and a way of compensating for perceived past misdeeds.

These men and women strive to place themselves in the larger moral cosmos. Their role in getting infected—even if accidental—conflicts with their need to see themselves as morally blameless. As a result they enter a particular place, no longer on the familiar moral terrain they had inhabited earlier. They now try to establish and justify in larger terms their actions and continued lives. They seek to do good and volunteer—not just as a way to achieve symbolic immortality but as a response to moral promptings.

On one hand these findings parallel those of Robert Jay Lifton in his studies of Hiroshima and Nagasaki. In both instances, individuals sought connections through family, religion, and "experiential transcendence" (i.e., through drugs and, to a lesser, more transient extent, sex).

Yet instructive differences arose as well. The men and women here seek to adapt not only to death but to a range of social problems. Death in America also differs from that in other cultures. In Japan, individuals more commonly sought connection to "nature"—the sense that trees and grass would continue around them even after they died. The atomic bomb had destroyed plants as well as humans, and fear spread that the bomb's effects on foliage might linger. Works of nature hold particular importance in Shinto beliefs and in traditional Japanese culture.

Nor did an exact equivalent of HIV-land arise in the situations Lifton described. Family and community played vital roles in the traditional Japanese culture that merely continued. But in HIV-land, many individuals, estranged from their families, look to create a new community to replace social networks now lost.

Numbness, found by Lifton among individuals directly affected by massive death, emerges from HIV more among the uninfected—the rest of society. Patients with HIV minimize or reconceptualize the disease, but rarely feel numb. A blood test that doesn't otherwise alter one's experience of one's body can easily fade from consciousness. Many individuals describe feeling "numb" only in the first few minutes or hours after testing positive, and then deal with the fact of infection in other ways— though some patients then minimize their infection. But widespread death from HIV induces numbness from the public at large who fall into indifference, pleased to hear of treatment advances but of little else concerning the epidemic. In short, HIV, while in some ways resembling other instances of massive death, also differs substantially, given in part the cultural context and public perceptions of the epidemic.

The Biology of the Self

HIV transformed lives far more than I had expected. In response to feelings of shame and the threat of death, individuals reexamined and remade their inner as well as outer worlds. Patients radically shifted their identities and purpose. George Sullivan and Wilma Smith, for example, came to embrace the illness and to refer to themselves, respectively, as "HIV George" and "HIV Wilma." In our identity-conscious age, self-definitions have become more fluid. Still, self-change, though necessary for personal growth, remains difficult. Successful people seem particularly good at it, yet HIV has impelled many otherwise seemingly ordinary men and women to grow in extraordinary ways.

HIV illustrates how notions of self become constructed and altered. Conversion experiences, in earlier centuries viewed in religious terms, can now result from illness. Changes in the outward body can affect the inner self as men and women make sense of their ailments and mortality. Infected men and women construct not only their illness but themselves as ill, seeing themselves not as patients but as part of a community through which they create an identity. Thus members of HIV-land prefer to be called PWAs instead of AIDS patients. They try to see HIV as a nondisease that affects nonpatients who are not "infected by" but are only "with" the virus.

Since the last century the self has been framed in psychological terms by Nietzsche, Freud, and others, and viewed as amenable to change through psychological interventions such as psychoanalysis. Recently, however, that paradigm has been challenged. Alterations in self brought about by pharmacologic agents such as

Prozac have been one part of this shift, but the stories presented here illustrate self-transformation occurring also as a result of disease. To become "HIV Wilma," for example, suggests the emergence of a new identity. The mechanisms may be psychological, but the impetus to change is biologic.

To adopt an identity because of a traumatic illness raises key questions about the parameters and definitions of self in the first place. Freud never addressed the notion of new identities forming out of social or medical upheavals. Yet the HIV epidemic offers evidence of such shifts. Illness, along with culture of origin and career, can profoundly shape self-concept in ways not examined by Freud.

At the same time HIV illustrates how culture frames and mediates such changes. HIV-land provides both a language and a social order for molding such new identities. Homosexual men, for example, in coming out as gay and as HIV positive, enter subcultures that then help influence everything from their styles of clothing and leisure activities to their anticipated life spans.

Yet not all aspects of such transformation are coveted. While former injecting drug users praise the beneficial aspects of being infected, many gay men dissent. Disease can raise or lower social status. Still, some gay men, such as Kerry Musgrove, report that after being "lost" much of their adulthood, HIV has helped them find purpose.

Although the lives of both gay men and drug users have often improved, differences clearly remain. Many gay men have struggled for decades in difficult fields, building careers that must now be abandoned. Yet even many of these men readily cite the lessons they have learned, the grace and wisdom they have attained, and the appreciation of aspects of life they have previously overlooked.

Voices

These men and women spoke far more openly and eloquently than I had anticipated. Drug users in particular I thought would be hard to get to know, and not necessarily sympathetic.

Yet these patients feel a need to speak. Many reported that participating in this project helped them by providing an opportunity to reflect on and make sense of their lives. The process of organizing a narrative of their experiences served an important function in coping with the virus. Robert Jay Lifton and others have described how elderly individuals tend to engage in a "life review," reminiscing over the past. HIV-infected individuals find such a process difficult, because they view as taboo the behaviors that had transmitted the illness. Death, moreover, has arrived too soon. It is difficult to achieve a sense of the completion of life while one is still young. Large uncertainties remain: death threatens even as new medications hold potential promise.

Yet through these tales runs what I call a "will to wholeness," a desire to put one's life together as a coherent story. Patients construct their experiences as narratives and employ narrative techniques and frameworks. Aaron, for instance, refers to the course of his illness as "a never-ending story." Individuals see a beginning, middle, and possible end. Events unfold. For many patients, past mistakes ultimately yield good—lessons learned or applied, high personal costs recompensed. Pain is transfigured into growth.

These narratives embody a logic, integrity, and organic flow. Forced to confront their potential demise, patients yielded up their lives to be heard, and expressed these issues better than I could. They now examined their lives more closely but also wanted somehow to contribute to others.

Their narratives convey, too, a sense of the fullness and complexity of their lives. For example, the epidemic now hits hardest inner-city women—such as Yvette, Dede, Gerry, and Olana—for whom HIV is not the major problem but one of several, along with poverty and homelessness. How these women deal with HIV and with the rest of their lives is of a piece, each set of issues affecting and reflecting the other. To understand the context of their lives, these women's own perspectives must be heard.

Through these narratives HIV also emerges as a cultural problem. Patients respond to their illness as a social as well as a personal crisis, and frame their situation not merely in individual but in communal and global terms. The epidemic exists in particular worlds and thus needs to be seen in a cultural, not just a medical or psychiatric, context.

Language is important here for other reasons. These men and women, creating an imaginary place—not the moral universe in which they were raised, but a new one both internally and externally—seek words that will describe and define. HIV-land helps propagate and promulgate this new discourse. These narratives reveal how a psychosocial problem gets conceptualized in new ways. Patients' views of HIV differ substantially, for example, from those of physicians. Clinicians, policymakers, and others can benefit from paying more attention to patients' own words and maintaining an open perspective.

I have tried to let these patients speak for themselves, to present their lives whole in order to bear witness and do justice to what I heard. I have sought to convey the force of these men and women's individuality, not merely reduce them to psychiatric categories. Some researchers may wish to classify these patients further, but an overreduction or oversimplification of their lives would do them a disservice.

By integrating psychiatry, social science, and close analyses of language and text, these individuals' experiences can be better understood than by using any one of these approaches alone. Social science illuminates the importance of community and social structures. Psychiatry illustrates how these patterns of response relate to mental health. Yet medical and psychological research have too readily removed themselves from the experiences of individual lives. Narratives give face and voice to the HIV epidemic, adding flesh and blood to statistics and rigid categories and concepts. The attention to narratives advocated in anthropology through the writings of Clifford Geertz and others has been essentially ignored by psychiatry, particularly in approaches to medical disease and AIDS. Behavioral HIV studies have generally relied on more quantitative cognitive-behavioral models, with structured questionnaires that examine segments of patients experiences (for example, counting depressive symptoms or interactions with family), separating rather than integrating these phenomena in order to understand the whole of an individual's experiences. Yet the language that people themselves use adds subtlety and depth, nuance and richness to an understanding of the psychological mechanisms at play.

Some readers may not like what these men and women report, particularly concerning minimization of the illness. Freud has written extensively on the process whereby the pointing out of psychological defenses elicits resistance. As one AIDS activist I spoke to about this data said, "What's wrong with denial? I like it." And the findings here regarding moral and spiritual issues may not be considered politically correct. But my objective has been to present what I discovered—the patterns people followed, and their advantages and disadvantages. I do not pass judgment. To understand the full range of responses to the illness is crucial to helping people adapt as effectively as possible.

New medications make these findings of ever increasing importance. I completed these interviews before the July 1996 International AIDS Conference in Vancouver, where the successes of protease inhibitors received wide attention for the first time. Yet

the extensive conversations I have had since then with HIV-
positive men and women have demonstrated that the patterns described here remain crucial. HIV continues to spread, yet the national death rate from AIDS has declined as people are living
longer with the virus. Thus more people face for longer periods
the challenges of adapting and finding meaning in their lives.
Many patients again look forward to the future; many who retired
now contemplate working. Still, problems persist—losses and
threats of death in oneself and others; uncertainty; stigma from
disease and from years of drug use; homosexuality; racism; and
poverty. People need not only medications but meaning. Scars of
past deaths and fears of future ones linger. New drugs help, but
they aren't enough. They offer the possibility of longer life but no
guarantees. For tens of thousands of people, these new medications have already failed. Thousands of patients lack the funds or
insurance to obtain these treatments, and many patients lead
chaotic and unscheduled lives that deter physicians from offering
the complicated regimens. Nor do physicians always prescribe the
new drugs correctly. Patients may relapse or encounter resistance,
become sicker, and again face more severe problems.

The media have rushed to see protease inhibitors as wonder
drugs but have been slower to report on these medications' difficulties. The new treatments have been viewed as though the AIDS
epidemic has been stopped, as if other vexing issues related to the
epidemic—arising from poverty, stigma, drug use, and despair—
were no longer problems. To what degree have these medications
been imbued with hype and magical powers? The anthropologist
Bronislaw Malinowski has written in *Magic, Science and Religion*
about similarities between magic and science. Both seek to provide
confidence in the face of uncertainty and fear, warding off demor-
alization, and both employ rituals. The sociologist Renée Fox, in
The Sociology of Medicine, has gone further in elaborating forms
of "scientific magic" whereby, for example, beneficial aspects of

new drugs are heralded initially, and only later tempered by the recognition of problems. Protease inhibitors offer enormous benefits, but attention to these other ongoing problems needs to continue as well. Still, these treatments have brought much hope to many. As the epidemic continues to evolve, the patterns presented here may change in some ways; yet I expect that essentially they will remain and help us make sense of responses to the virus.

The Health of America

HIV raises in bold relief issues that each of us will one day confront. We will all face death, though we rarely think about it. Yet as it grows older the American population is becoming increasingly concerned about illness, health, and mortality. Those with HIV—mostly baby boomers—have had to face these issues before others of their generation, and have illustrated what does and does not impede and help. Even former atheists and agnostics I talked with locate their own conceptual frameworks for coming to terms with spiritual ideas, whether these frameworks are abstract or scientifically based. Their responses illuminate how death and dying are handled among people of different backgrounds, including gay men and the poor, who seek to transcend mortality and prejudice no differently than do others. Yet their options and resources vary.

This study has special implications for patients with disorders other than HIV. The sick in general face stigma, fear, and isolation. These HIV-infected men and women offer new ways of addressing these problems. For example, HIV sets new precedents for the social organization of patients. On one hand HIV-land parallels the formation of "clubs" of people who are sick, as found in Renée Fox's study of patients on a renal research ward, described in her book *Experiment Perilous*. Yet the HIV community has pushed the limits of such social structures. Patients with other illnesses have consciously begun to adopt many of the mechanisms of HIV-land, joining in groups to fight for themselves. Thus there are now PWLs, People with Lupus, in the same way there are PWAs. Such organizations have seen the advantages of altering the terms by which patients are perceived by others—and in turn may view themselves. The effectiveness of AIDS activism has politically inspired patients with other disorders. If government cutbacks in health care continue, patient advocacy will gain added importance as competition for limited funds grows.

Indeed, never before in America has a disease become the basis of a political movement. The radical methods employed by some in the HIV community—taking to the streets—result in part from the threat of death. Larry Kramer, when he started ACT-UP, told a roomful of gay men in New York City, "Half of you will be dead in seven years." That realization mobilized the group. They had less to lose than they would have otherwise. In retrospect, the threat of death in Vietnam galvanized much of 1960s radicalism in ways that historians who follow politics alone still underappreciate.

Politics and death are intricately connected. Political decisions influence the lives and deaths of patients through research budgets and social services. Conversely, political activism provides a mode of symbolic immortality, a way of benefiting other patients in the future. Although not all PWAs politicize their illness, those who do gain a means not only of affecting the future but of voicing otherwise unexpressed frustration and rage.

Future epidemics will no doubt arise. Disease outbreaks have beset man since he first evolved; social and environmental changes continually create new niches for infectious agents. Man and parasites fight a ceaseless war, and the latter seize any opportunity for advantage. Now, greater travel between previously isolated areas generates further opportunities for germs to spread to new locales. Urban areas and populations of injecting drug users and gay men are particularly vulnerable, given behaviors that can potentially transmit infection. These groups, still in social and behavioral transition, have not fully developed defenses and immunities against parasites and viruses. Indeed, recent years have witnessed urban outbreaks not only of HIV but of herpes, hepatitis, and tuberculosis.

Yet epidemics that devastate many regions of the world have not appeared in the West in the past sixty years, during a time when depth psychology and social science have begun to investigate the meanings of death and dying. Now these perspectives can be brought to bear. To document and examine these men's and women's lives will help others understand the responses of our own time and place to this modern plague.

HIV has also impelled American medicine and psychiatry to confront several biases. Racism, homophobia, Calvinistic attitudes toward drug use, and what I call "anti-AIDSism"—a distancing and distaste for the virus and what it represents—still infect these professions. In addition, modern medicine and psychiatry, trying to uphold themselves as purely scientific, look askance at spirituality. Psychoanalysts from Freud onward have regarded spiritual ideas as mere "illusions," the products of defenses. As a scientist it is easy to be suspicious of spiritual ideas. But many of the men and women in this book *believe*. Spirituality can clearly help individuals with HIV and other diseases. Medicine can delay but never eliminate death; spirituality provides compensation. Yet spirituality, part of an individual's private world, is rarely if ever discussed socially. Each of us clearly lives with it, but not in daily conversation.

This study has wider implications for psychotherapy too, demonstrating the psychological benefits of activities (such as spirituality and volunteerism) not ordinarily prescribed as psychotherapeutic. Patients and their caregivers and loved ones should be aware of the patterns presented here as options, along with the possible risks. Involvement in HIV-land, beliefs in a higher power, work and volunteerism, and strengthened connections with kin can support individuals in vital ways. To reframe the illness helps many but also has disadvantages. Substance abuse, though often temporarily allaying patients' concerns, can also be problematic.

Surely we need more psychosocial research on HIV. Billions of government research dollars have failed to discover a definitive cure or effective vaccine to stop the epidemic's continued rise. Despite the development of new medications for those already infected, additional support is still necessary to understand and overcome barriers to prevention and the further spread of HIV in the first place. Yet the most effective prevention campaign for adolescents, for example, was identified through research several years ago, and used street theater. The program was so successful that it was defunded, because it had been financed as a research study, not as a program to be implemented. The strictly scientific question had been answered: the program was found to work. Similarly the Bush administration several years ago initiated an information program called America Responds to AIDS. Television ads announced it and provided an 800 number. Yet only one of ten calls was ever answered—all that funding would allow. It was more important to claim that America was responding than actually to provide a response. Psychosocial research has been similarly limited in scope and funding, but the issues involved are complex and ignored only at our peril. These narratives have suggested, for example, that how individuals view their illness affects the likelihood they will transmit it to others. And the barriers to prevention, as shown here, can be enormous and must be carefully addressed.

These patients' experiences also cry out with questions of whether and how to improve social policies. Health care, poverty, racism, and homophobia now receive increased legislative attention at national, state, and local levels. The accounts presented here illustrate the impact of policies in these areas on individual lives and the challenges that legislation on drug use, poverty, and crime face—how deeply entrenched these problems remain, particularly as social services are reduced.

Recently a National Institutes of Health council evaluated all AIDS prevention studies conducted to date. An overwhelming finding: social and legislative resistance to putting into practice insights gained from research. Prejudice against gays, the poor, and people with AIDS persists. There is still a long way to go to overcome deep-seated social indifference and hate. These tales demonstrate how such attitudes harm people, and at the same time how individuals try to adapt and make sense of such difficulties.

Even if AIDS is eventually cured, these examples of endurance, insight, and courage will continue on.

Index

A NOTE ON THE AUTHOR

Robert Klitzman is assistant professor of clinical psychiatry at Columbia University. Born in New York City, he received a bachelor's degree from Princeton University and an M.D. from Yale. In two earlier books about his medical and psychiatric training, *A Year-long Night* and *In a House of Dreams and Glass*, Dr. Klitzman won acclaim for his honest, perceptive, and compassionate portrayal of the making of a physician. Among several honors, he has been a Robert Wood Johnson Foundation Clinical Scholar, a Burroughs-Wellcome Fellow, and a Merck Company Foundation Fellow at Yaddo. He lives in New York City.